# Practical
# Neuro-Oncology

D1568495

# Practical
# Neuro-Oncology
## A Guide to Patient Care

Leslie D. McAllister, M.D.

*Clinical Assistant Professor of Medicine, Division
of Hematology–Oncology, Oregon Health Sciences
University, Portland; Clinical Director of Legacy Brain
and Spinal Cord Tumor Program, Good Samaritan
Hospital, Portland*

John H. Ward, M.D.

*Professor of Medicine and Chief of Oncology Division,
University of Utah School of Medicine, Salt Lake City;
Medical Director, Huntsman Cancer Institute at the
University of Utah, Salt Lake City*

Susan F. Schulman, B.A., C.C.R.A.

*Program Coordinator of Translational Screening,
University of Utah School of Medicine, Salt Lake City*

Lisa M. DeAngelis, M.D.

*Professor of Neurology, Weill Medical College of Cornell
University, New York; Chairman of Neurology, Memorial
Sloan-Kettering Cancer Center, New York*

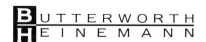

Boston   Oxford   Auckland   Johannesburg   Melbourne   New Delhi

**Library of Congress Cataloging-in-Publication Data**

Practical neuro-oncology : a guide to patient care / Leslie D. McAllister . . . [et al.].
   p. ; cm.
  Includes bibliographical references and index.
  ISBN 0-7506-7180-7 (pbk. : alk. paper)
  1. Central nervous system—Cancer. I. McAllister, Leslie D.
  [DNLM: 1. Central Nervous System Neoplasms—therapy. WL 358 P896 2002]
  RC280.N43 P73 2000
  616.99'48—dc21

                            2001035367

**British Library Cataloguing-in-Publication Data**

A catalogue record for this book is available from the British Library.

The publisher offers special discounts on bulk orders of this book.
For information, please contact:

    Manager of Special Sales
    Butterworth–Heinemann
    225 Wildwood Avenue
    Woburn, MA 01801-2041
    Tel: 781-904-2500
    Fax: 781-904-2620

For information on all Butterworth–Heinemann publications available, contact our World Wide Web home page at: http://www.bh.com

10 9 8 7 6 5 4 3 2 1

Printed in the United States of America

*This book is dedicated to our patients
and their loved ones.*

# Contents

# Preface

Cancer is a major cause of death and disability in the United States. It is the second leading cause of death for people of all ages, and is the leading cause of death for people ages 35–64. Neurologic complications are common and becoming more prevalent as treatment for systemic malignancy improves survival for many cancer patients. The central nervous system (CNS) has long been described as a sanctuary site, where tumor cells can propagate in tissue that is largely inaccessible to the chemotherapy regimens that successfully treat systemic tumors. This sanctuary site serves as a protected environment for metastatic cells to grow and develop into clinically important lesions. In addition, some primary brain tumors are increasing in incidence, particularly among older patients and children. Primary brain tumors are an important cause of death and disability and often strike individuals in the prime of their lives.

Neurologic dysfunction from either primary or metastatic brain tumors is feared by patients and physicians alike because it compromises the patient's sense of self and also severely impairs the patient's level of independent function. Neurologic impairment not only shortens life but also markedly reduces the patient's quality of life. While many physicians have a nihilistic view of CNS involvement by cancer, early diagnosis and vigorous treatment can often prolong life and substantially improve or preserve the patient's neurologic function.

The goals of this book are (1) to provide basic knowledge about primary and metastatic brain tumors and nonmetastatic neurologic complications in cancer patients, (2) to review the clinical approach and diagnostic procedures in patients suspected of an intracranial tumor, and (3) to provide practical information regarding common clinical problems that occur in neuro-oncologic patients. This monograph is not intended to deliver a comprehensive discussion of each of these areas. For that, several recent monographs are available. However, it is our intention to highlight and discuss the common medical problems that arise in these patients and how non-neuro-oncologists might begin to deal with them. Given the increasing incidence of these problems, it is likely that many physicians will care for patients with brain tumors or neurologic complications of cancer. We do not intend this book to replace the need for consultation with specialists who are expert and experienced in dealing with these problems but rather to serve as a guide to the generalist who often makes the initial diagnosis and shares the care of these patients throughout their illness with a specialist.

*L. D. M.*

*J. H. W.*

*S. F. S.*

*L. M. D.*

# I

# General
# Information

# 1

# Primary Tumors of the Central Nervous System

This chapter provides general information regarding the types of primary tumors involving the brain and spinal cord and their relative frequencies and locations. Primary brain tumors can occur at any age, from infancy to late in life, and often afflict people during their prime years. Factors such as age, tumor location, and clinical presentation are helpful in differential diagnosis. A detailed discussion of the classifications and grading of brain tumors is beyond the scope of this book. An overview is presented here with selected references. More than half of newly diagnosed intracranial tumors are metastatic.

## Primary Brain Tumors

### Incidence and Statistics

- The annual combined incidence for all types of primary brain tumors is 11.5/100,000 person-years.
- The overall incidence of gliomas appears to be increasing, especially in the elderly. The explanation for this trend remains unclear.
- The overall incidence of primary brain tumors is higher in men (12.1/ 100,000 person-years) than women (11.0/100,000 person-years) and higher in whites than in blacks.
- Most types of primary brain tumors are more common in men with the exception of meningiomas, which are more common in women.

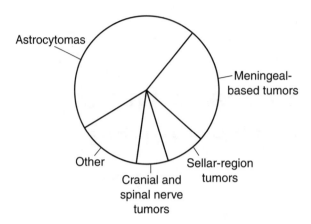

**Figure 1-1**    Pie chart illustrating the relative incidence of primary brain tumors. (Data from CBTRUS (2000) Statistical Report. Primary Brain Tumors in the United States, 1992–1997.)

Figure 1-1 illustrates the relative incidence of the more common primary brain tumors based on recently published data from the Central Brain Tumor Registry of the United States (CBTRUS).

## Location and Patient Age Determine Differential Diagnosis

- Specific tumor types tend to occur in typical locations in the nervous system.
- Specific tumor types tend to occur in certain age groups.
- Certain combinations of age and location provide distinct diagnostic and prognostic information. For example, the cerebellar astrocytoma of childhood and early adulthood has a more benign prognosis than astrocytomas located in the cerebral hemispheres in adulthood.

Table 1-1 lists the more common primary brain tumors by general locations for adults and children. These are broad generalizations, and the less common tumor types are not listed.

## Classification of Primary Brain Tumors

The classification of primary central nervous system (CNS) tumors has undergone frequent revision over the past several decades, as more is learned about the behavior and biology of these tumors. The reader is referred to the texts listed at the end of this chapter for brain tumor classifications. Not all pathologists use the same classification system. Nonetheless,

**Table 1-1**   Common Primary Brain Tumors in Adults and Children
by General Location

|  | *Adults* | *Children* |
|---|---|---|
| Supratentorial | Astrocytomas (all grades)<br>Meningiomas | Primitive neuroectodermal<br>tumors<br>Astrocytomas |
| Infratentorial | Acoustic neuroma<br>Ependymoma<br>Brain stem glioma | Cerebellar astrocytoma<br>Cerebellar medulloblastoma<br>Fourth ventricle ependymoma<br>Brain stem glioma |
| Pineal region and<br>third ventricle | Pineoblastoma<br>Germ cell tumors | Pineoblastoma<br>Germ cell tumors |
| Sellar and<br>parasellar | Pituitary adenoma<br>Craniopharyngioma<br>Meningioma | Craniopharyngioma<br>Optic nerve and chiasm gliomas |

under all systems, most tumor names relate to the putative cell of origin. For
example, astrocytomas arise from astrocytes.

## Primary Spinal Cord Tumors

- Tumor location with respect to the spinal cord and surrounding struc-
  tures is an important diagnostic factor.
- Tumor location-related categories are termed
  - Intramedullary
  - Intradural/extramedullary
  - Extradural
- In general, primary spinal cord tumors tend to be intramedullary or
  intradural/extramedullary, whereas metastatic spinal cord tumors
  tend to involve the epidural space and vertebral elements.

## Suggested Reading

Bigner DD, McLendon RE, Bruner JM (eds). *Russell and Rubinstein's Pathology of Tumors of the Nervous System* (6th ed). New York: Oxford University Press, 1998.

Burger PC, Scheithauer BW. *Atlas of Tumor Pathology: Tumors of the Central
Nervous System*. Third Series. Fascicle 10. Bethesda, MD: Armed Forces
Institute of Pathology, 1993.

Kleihues P, Burger PC, Scheithauer BW, Zülch KJ. *Histological Typing of Tumours of the Central Nervous System* (2nd ed). Berlin: Springer-Verlag, 1993.

Poirier J, Gray F, Escourolle R. *Manual of Basic Neuropathology* (3rd ed). Philadelphia: W.B. Saunders, 1990.

Surawicz TS, McCarthy BJ, Kupelian V, et al. Descriptive epidemiology of primary brain and CNS tumors: Results from the Central Brain Tumor Registry of the United States, 1990–1994. *Neuro-oncology.* 1999;1(1):14–25.

# 2

# Metastatic Tumors of the Central Nervous System

Metastasis to the central nervous system (CNS) is an important and common cause of neurologic symptoms in cancer patients. Direct metastasis to the brain, skull, and spine are the most common neurologic complications of cancer. Furthermore, neurologic symptoms are the initial symptoms of a tumor outside the nervous system in about 10% of cancer patients. The symptoms associated with nervous system metastasis significantly alter the quality of life of affected patients. The occurrence of CNS metastasis generally is considered by both patient and physician to signify treatment failure and patients with CNS metastasis typically have been excluded from most oncology clinical trials. Nonetheless, patients with CNS metastasis can benefit from therapies that are either tumor specific or palliative. Furthermore, specific therapy for some metastatic tumors can reduce symptoms and extend survival. Clinical trials for patients with CNS metastases are becoming more widely available as more effective treatments for systemic cancers have improved survival. This chapter discusses the types of nervous system metastases that develop.

## Spread of Cancer to the Central Nervous System

Cancer spreads to the nervous system by direct invasion, compression, or metastasis. Direct invasion or compression from contiguous tissues relates to the proximity of the nervous system to other structures, such as the brachial plexus, lumbosacral plexus, vertebral neuroforamina, base of skull, cranium, and pelvic bones. Metastasis to the CNS occurs via the hematogenous route or from the lymphatics, dural sinuses, or venous structures. These sites of involvement are listed in Table 2-1 along with some typical clinical examples. One or more metastatic sites can exist within an individual patient.

**Table 2-1**    Sites of Nervous System Involvement by Systemic Tumors

| Site of Involvement | Common Examples | Comments |
| --- | --- | --- |
| **Intracranial metastasis** | | |
| Brain parenchyma | Breast, lung, melanoma | |
| Pituitary gland | Breast, melanoma, germ cell, any site | |
| Dural based | Lung, prostate, breast | May be associated with effusion |
| Leptomeningeal disease | Breast, lung | |
| **Skull** | | |
| Skull base | Breast, prostate, osteosarcoma of skull, head and neck cancers | Usually symptomatic |
| Calvarium | Breast, prostate | Usually asymptomatic |
| **Spine** | | |
| Epidural | Lung, breast, prostate | Direct extension from vertebral body |
| | Neuroblastoma, lymphoma | Invasion of neuroforamina by paravertebral tumors |
| | Leukemia, lymphoma | Hematogenous |
| Leptomeningeal | Breast, lung | |
| Intramedullary | Breast, colon, lung, prostate | Rare but increasing |
| **Brachial plexus** | Lung, breast, lymphoma | Primary or metastasis in superior sulcus of lung or metastatic lymph nodes in axilla |
| **Lumbosacral plexus/sciatic nerve** | Pelvic tumors, metastasis in lymph nodes, metastasis in pelvic bones | |

## Intracranial Metastasis

Intracranial metastasis occurs to brain parenchyma, dural structures, or the leptomeninges.

### Brain Metastasis

Hematogenous spread is the most common mode of brain parenchymal metastasis, because the brain is richly vascularized and receives 20% of the cardiac output. Tumors from any site in the body can spread to the brain by this mode. Brain metastases often are accompanied by other systemic metastases, particularly to the lungs, although in some cases the brain is the only apparent site of metastasis. Brain metastasis can be single or multiple and involve any portion of the brain. Hematogenous metastases tend to deposit near the gray/white junction or in the "watershed" areas between large blood vessel circulations (anterior and middle cerebral arteries or middle cerebral artery and posterior cerebral artery). Although hematogenous metastases usually are microscopic, they can be larger and present as overt tumor emboli, causing abrupt neurologic symptoms in a stroke-like manner. Although brain metastases can originate from any primary tumor, certain primary tumors are more prone to metastasize to the brain, such as lung, breast, and melanoma.

- Hematogenous brain metastases usually are distributed proportionally by blood flow: 90% cerebrum and 10% posterior fossa.
- 50% of patients with brain metastases have single lesions.
- 20% of patients with brain metastases have two lesions.
- 10% of patients with brain metastases have more than five lesions.
- Pelvic primary tumors, such as those in the prostate, uterus, and gastrointestinal tracts, tend to metastasize to the posterior fossa more often than other primary tumors: pelvic and gastrointestinal tumors, 53% posterior fossa and 47% cerebrum.
- Unusual causes of brain metastases include ovarian cancer, sarcomas, prostate cancer, and thyroid cancer.

### Dural Metastasis

Metastasis to dural structures generally occurs by hematogenous spread or direct invasion from a contiguous bone. These metastases sometimes are associated with effusions and radiographic and clinical findings similar to that of a subdural hygroma. In other cases, the tumor mimics a meningioma radiographically. Dural metastases can invade the underlying brain and cause focal edema and associated neurologic symptoms. Because of their cortical location, these processes tend to cause seizures early in the course.

### *Leptomeningeal Metastasis*

Metastasis to the leptomeninges is an uncommon but well-recognized clinical presentation in cancer patients. Leptomeningeal metastasis most commonly is due to breast, lung, or melanoma primary tumors. Leptomeningeal involvement also occurs with the hematologic malignancies, particularly non-Hodgkin's lymphoma. Diagnosis and treatment are discussed in Chapter 29.

### Skull Metastasis

Metastases to the skull are divided into two categories by general site: calvarium and skull base. Metastases to the calvarium usually are asymptomatic. When symptoms do occur, they relate to tumor growth compressing the underlying brain or an associated subdural effusion. Metastases to the skull base quickly become symptomatic because of their proximity to cranial nerves and vascular structures. Syndromes related to skull-based tumors are discussed in Chapter 34.

### Spinal Metastasis

The spine most often is affected by metastatic disease involving the epidural space. This usually occurs as direct tumor spread from a vertebral body (85%) or by invasion of paravertebral masses through a neuroforamin (10–15%). True hematogenous spread of tumor to the epidural space is uncommon and generally limited to patients with lymphoreticular malignancies. Intramedullary spinal metastases are rare, usually associated with brain metastases, and probably occur by hematogenous spread.

### Suggested Reading

Bigner DD, McLendon RE, Bruner JM (eds). *Russell and Rubinstein's Pathology of Tumors of the Nervous System* (6th ed). New York: Oxford University Press, 1998.
DeAngelis LM. Management of brain metastases. *Cancer Invest.* 1994;12(2): 156–165.

# 3

# Genetic Syndromes and Risk Factors

Although the large majority of primary brain and spinal cord tumors are sporadic, several genetic syndromes increase the risk. There is a low, but statistically significant, increased risk for developing a brain tumor if a first-degree relative has been diagnosed with glioma. The explanation for this remains unclear. There are no clearly identified nongenetic risk factors for most primary brain tumors.

## Genetic Syndromes

The genetic syndromes associated with primary brain tumors are summarized in Table 3-1. If a genetic syndrome is suspected, a genetic counselor can provide instructions about genetic testing and counseling for the patient and family members. The National Society of Genetic Counselors (610-872-7608; www.nsgc.org) can provide a referral for the counselor closest to the patient's home. If distance prohibits the patient from visiting a genetic counselor, the society can provide information about shipping blood specimens and detailing the family history.

**Table 3-1**  Hereditary Syndromes Associated with Tumors of the Nervous System

| Hereditary Condition | Type of CNS Tumor | Chromosome Involved | Gene Involved[a] | Gene Product |
|---|---|---|---|---|
| Neurofibromatosis type 1 (von Recklinghausen's disease, peripheral NF[b]) | Optic nerve glioma, pilocytic astrocytoma, cerebellar astrocytoma, anaplastic astrocytoma, glioblastoma multiforme, ependymoma, meningioma, plexiform neurofibroma, peripheral nerve sheath sarcoma, ganglioneuroma, pheochromocytoma | 17q11.2 | NF1 | Neurofibromin |
| Neurofibromatosis type 2 (bilateral acoustic NF, central NF) | Schwannoma, meningioma, ependymoma | 22q12.2 | NF2 | Merlin (also known as schwannomin) |
| Tuberous sclerosis | Subependymal giant-cell astrocytoma, ependymoma, astrocytic glioma, ganglioneuroma, glioblastoma | 9q 34 16p13.3 12q22-q24.2 | TSC1 TSC2 TSC3 | Tuberin |
| von Hippel-Lindau disease | Hemangioblastoma of CNS and eye | 3p25-26 | VHL | VHL protein |
| Li-Fraumeni syndrome | Glioma, medulloblastoma, ependymoma, choroid plexus tumor | 17p13.1 | TP53 | p53 |
| Familial adenomatous polyposis (Turcot's and Gardner's syndromes) | Brain tumors of diverse histologic types, including glioblastoma and medulloblastoma | 5q21-22 | APC | APC protein |

| | | | | |
|---|---|---|---|---|
| Hereditary nonpolyposis colorectal cancer syndrome | Brain tumors of diverse histologic types, including glioblastoma and medulloblastoma | 3p22-23<br>2p16<br>2q31-33<br>7p22 | *MLH1*<br>*MLH2*<br>*PMS1*<br>*PMS2* | Mismatch repair enzymes |
| Nevoid basal-cell carcinoma syndrome (Gorlin's syndrome) | Medulloblastoma | 19q22.1-q22.3 | *NBCCS* | Putative transmembrane protein |
| Cowden disease | Meningioma and medulloblastoma | 10q22-q23 | *MHAM* | Not yet identified |
| MEN[b] | | | | |
|   Type 1 | Parathyroid adenoma, pancreatic islet cell tumor, pituitary adenoma, carcinoid | 11q13 | Unknown | |
|   Type 2A | Pheochromocytoma, parathyroid hyperplasia, medullary carcinoma of thyroid | 10q11.2 | *RET* | |
|   Type 2B | Gastrointestinal ganglioneuroma, medullary carcinoma of thyroid, pheochromocytoma, oral and ocular neuroma | 10q11.2 | *RET* | |
| FMTC[b] | Medullary carcinoma of thyroid | 10q11.2 | *RET* | |
| Retinoblastoma deletion syndrome | Retinoblastoma, pineoblastoma | 13q14.2 | *RB1* | RB protein |
| Carney's complex | | | Unknown | |
| Bannayan's syndrome | Retinoblastoma, pineoblastoma | | Unknown | |

CNS, central nervous system.

[a]From GDB™ genome database (1990). Inheritance of all syndromes is autosomally dominant.

[b]NF, neurofibromatosis; MEN, multiple endocrine neoplasia; FMTC, familial medullary thyroid carcinoma.

Reprinted with permission from McLendon RE, Tien RD. Genetic syndromes associated with tumors and/or hamartomas. In DD Bigner, RE McLendon, JM Bruner (eds). *Russell and Rubinstein's Pathology of Tumors of the Nervous System* (6th ed). New York: Oxford University Press, 1998:373.

## Nongenetic Risk Factors

### Occupational and Environmental

Few issues in medicine are as potentially contentious as the suspicion of environmental and occupational causes of cancer, including brain tumors.

Prior cranial irradiation is the only risk factor that definitely predisposes to brain tumor formation. The following list of possible risk factors is not intended to draw conclusions about causes of an individual patient's tumor. Rather, it is a compilation of suggestive epidemiological studies, some of which are not confirmed by other studies. This point should be emphasized if a patient provides a reference implicating a specific occupational or environmental factor.

- Ionizing radiation: prior cranial radiation for another disease, atomic bomb exposure, work in the nuclear industry. Therapeutic radiation is a well-defined risk factor for meningiomas, astrocytomas, and sarcomas.
- Nonionizing radiation: electromagnetic fields, radiofrequency radiation such as microwave exposure, radar equipment, amateur radio operator exposure, telecommunications worker exposure, utility worker exposure, cellular phones.
- Nitrosamines: cosmetics, automobile interiors, rubber, drugs containing these compounds.
- Industrial chemicals: vinyl chloride, petrochemicals, formaldehyde, organochlorines, inorganic mercury, glycerol polyglycidyl ether, and organic solvents.

### Other Possible Risk Factors

None of these factors have been conclusively implicated in brain tumor development but have been suggested by some studies. Many are the subject of conflicting reports.

- Social class: higher in upper classes.
- Religion: Jewish, Mormon.
- Community setting: rural vs. urban, "cancer clusters" in specific residential areas.
- Specific regions of the United States: Minnesota.
- Other countries: Scandinavia, Israel, United Kingdom.
- Dietary factors: high serum cholesterol, use of vegetable fats, smoking, alcohol, and cured meats.

- Viruses or virus-like particles:
  - HIV disease, or any chronic immunosuppressed state, is a risk factor for primary CNS lymphoma.
  - Other considerations have included simian virus 40 and other polyoma viruses, nonpolyoma viruses such as cytomegalovirus and herpes, the poliomyelitis vaccine, and *Toxoplasma gondii*.
- Infections: during pregnancy (for infant brain tumors).
- Trauma: head trauma, perinatal trauma, acoustic trauma.
- Hormonal factors: steroids, progesterones.
- Pre-existing medical conditions: history of seizures, childhood exposure to barbiturates, kidney transplant, primary hyperthyroidism, multiple sclerosis.

Identification of patterns that could be relevant to both genetic and nongenetic risk factors remains an intriguing scientific issue. If an incidence cluster or family group that might be of interest is observed, the observation should be reported.

## Suggested Reading

Bigner DD, McLendon RE, and Bruner JM (eds). *Russell and Rubinstein's Pathology of Tumors of the Nervous System* (6th ed). New York: Oxford University Press, 1998.

Rom WN. *Environmental and Occupational Medicine* (3rd ed). Philadelphia: Lippincott-Raven, 1998.

# II

# Initial Patient Evaluation and Care

# 4

# Brain Tumor Presentations

Signs and symptoms due to an intracranial mass lesion can be localizing, nonlocalizing, or falsely localizing. For example, headache is nonlocalizing and is a common presenting symptom of an intracranial mass lesion. In general, the signs and symptoms due to intracranial mass lesions depend on their location in the nervous system, size, and growth rate, rather than the specific type of tumor. Symptoms usually are progressive in nature, unless the presenting symptom is a seizure. Patients with primary brain tumors rarely manifest constitutional symptoms, such as weight loss, fever and chills, or night sweats. Patients with metastatic tumors of the nervous system may have signs and symptoms related to their primary tumor outside the nervous system.

## Signs and Symptoms

Table 4-1 lists the three potential types of signs and symptoms associated with intracranial mass lesions. Localizing signs and symptoms are those that relate directly to the location of the mass in the nervous system and are of localizing diagnostic value, such as hemiparesis. Nonlocalizing signs and symptoms, such as lethargy, are those that relate to increased intracranial pressure and generalized brain dysfunction due to cerebral edema, ventricular obstruction, or venous sinus obstruction. False localizing signs and symptoms are those that could lead to an incorrect localization, such as a cranial nerve (CN) VI palsy.

In general, patients with primary brain tumors or single metastatic tumors can present with any of these signs and symptoms, whereas patients with multiple brain metastases tend to present with generalized symptoms

**Table 4-1**    Signs and Symptoms in Patients with Brain Tumors

| Category | Mechanisms | Examples |
|---|---|---|
| Localizing | Focal brain irritation<br>Focal brain dysfunction | Partial seizures<br>Aphasia<br>Contralateral sensory loss<br>Contralateral weakness<br>Visual field deficits |
| Nonlocalizing | Increased intracranial pressure<br>Dural sinus obstruction<br>Hydrocephalus | Headaches<br>Nausea or vomiting<br>Confusion → stupor → coma<br>Personality or attention changes<br>Memory loss<br>Loss of balance<br>Papilledema |
| False localizing | Increased intracranial pressure<br>Bifrontal tumor involvement<br>Uncal herniation | Horizontal diplopia (CN VI palsy)<br>"Frontal ataxia"<br>Ipsilateral hemiparesis |

and may lack localizing findings. Tumors tend to be diagnosed early—when they are relatively small—either when they are associated with seizures or located in critical regions of the central nervous system (CNS), including the motor cortex, language cortex, afferent visual pathways, or brain stem. Tumors tend to be diagnosed late—when they are relatively large—when they are slow growing or affect clinically "silent" portions of the brain. For example, a frontal lobe tumor, especially when slow growing, can reach a relatively large size before producing symptoms. Parietal/occipital lobe tumors, particularly in the nondominant hemisphere, also can reach a large size prior to diagnosis because the patient does not notice the associated visual field loss or apraxias due to the phenomenon of "neglect." Recognizing that a patient has symptoms related to a possible brain tumor is important, because the neurologic examination is sometimes normal or only minimally abnormal in patients with structural lesions. Table 4-2 lists some common symptom constellations and their associated localization in the CNS.

Several clinical features warrant special comment:

- Seizures (partial or generalized) are the presenting symptom in 15–20% of patients with intracranial tumors. Seizures occur in up to 50% of patients with melanoma metastases, oligodendrogliomas, and tumors that have a hemorrhagic component. Seizures also are more common with cortically based tumors.
- Seizures are much less common in patients with infratentorial tumors than in those with supratentorial tumors.

**Table 4-2**  Syndromes Associated with Tumors by Location and Typical Examples

| Syndrome | Localization | Examples of Tumor Type |
|---|---|---|
| Obstructing hydrocephalus:<br>  Headache<br>  Nausea or vomiting<br>  Confusion or ataxia | Posterior fossa tumor | Cerebellar astrocytoma<br>Medulloblastoma<br>Fourth ventricle ependymoma |
| Brain stem signs and<br>  symptoms, alert, intact<br>  cognition | Brain stem | Brain stem glioma |
| Foster Kennedy syndrome:<br>  Unilateral visual loss<br>  Contralateral papilledema | Sphenoid ridge | Meningioma |
| Parinaud's syndrome:<br>  Light-near pupillary<br>    dissociation<br>  Impaired upgaze<br>  Retraction convergence<br>    nystagmus<br>  Quadraparesis (late) | Compression or<br>  involvement of<br>  tectal plate | Pineal region tumor<br>Tectal plate glioma |
| Hemichorea | Basal ganglia | Astrocytoma, lymphoma |
| Frontal lobe syndrome:<br>  Gait apraxia<br>  Incontinence<br>  Memory loss<br>  Affective changes | Bifrontal tumor or<br>  unilateral tumor<br>  with compression<br>  of contralateral<br>  frontal lobe | Astrocytoma<br>Meningioma<br>Lymphoma |

- "Stroke-like" onset of symptoms usually is due to hemorrhage within the tumor or, less commonly, macroscopic tumor embolus from systemic cancer.
- Although intratumoral hemorrhage can occur in any primary or metastatic brain tumor, certain tumors have a greater tendency to bleed, including metastasis from melanoma, choriocarcinoma, and thyroid cancer and the primary brain tumors glioblastoma and oligodendroglioma.
- Because lung cancer is the most common cause of brain metastases, it is the most common metastasis associated with hemorrhage.

## Neurologic Examination

The neurologic exam is useful in identifying deficits of which the patient is unaware, such as focal weakness, cognitive difficulties, or upper quadrant visual deficits. A careful exam also can elucidate the specific neuroanatomic localization of symptoms. The patient's history often is sufficient to suggest an intracranial mass, and diagnostic evaluation should proceed accordingly.

- Patients with new onset of seizures should have an enhanced magnetic resonance imaging (MRI) scan of the brain to exclude an intracranial tumor. The clinical information should be transmitted to the radiologist performing the scan to optimize the diagnostic value of the study.
- A normal or minimally abnormal neurologic exam or the absence of papilledema does not exclude an intracranial mass.
- Some patients with brain tumors initially are misdiagnosed as having strokes. However, their clinical presentation rarely is that of a typical stroke, since brain tumor symptoms usually are subacute in onset and progressive.
- Beware of the diagnosis of sinusitis particularly when there are
  - Associated neurologic symptoms.
  - Severe headaches.
  - No signs of sinusitis on imaging (computed tomography [CT] scan of sinuses).
  - One or more antibiotic failures.
  - Recurrent or progressive symptoms in the absence of fever.
- Headache presentations that raise suspicion for an intracranial mass include
  - "Brain tumor" headaches: headaches that awaken the patient from sleep (with the exception of cluster headache), morning headaches (patient wakes up with headache), vomiting that is not preceded by nausea or is projectile, headache that increases with Valsalva or other maneuvers that increase intracranial pressure (ICP).
  - New-onset headaches in an older patient or a change in headache pattern in a patient with chronic headaches.
  - Persistent headaches at any age that do not respond to nonsteroidal anti-inflammatory drugs or weak opioids or are associated with nausea and vomiting.
  - Migraines with persistent neurologic deficit or an "aura" that persists during the headache.
  - Although frontal headaches can occur in patients with sinusitis, they are not associated with neurologic symptoms or symptoms of increased ICP.
  - Dementia or personality change in a young adult should raise suspicion for an intracranial mass. The development of apathy and withdrawal often are attributed to depression, especially in older patients but frequently are the first symptoms of a brain tumor.

- A small percentage of patients with primary brain tumors present with fever; the mechanism for this is poorly understood.

## Suggested Reading

Posner JB. *Neurologic Complications of Cancer.* Philadelphia: F.A. Davis, 1995.

Schold SC Jr, Burger PC, Mendelsohn DB, et al. *Primary Tumors of the Brain and Spinal Cord.* Boston: Butterworth–Heinemann, 1997.

# 5

# Spinal Cord Tumor Presentations

Suspected spinal cord involvement is an emergency situation because timely diagnosis and management affects neurologic outcome. The presentation of a tumor in or around the spinal cord depends on its location—epidural, intradural and extra-medullary, or intramedullary. Along with this, the level of the spinal cord affected helps localize the process and direct neuro-imaging studies. The most common location for a spinal cord tumor is epidural. Epidural tumor is generally metastatic and usually presents with pain. Signs and symptoms of spinal cord compression follow in some patients. The most common sources of epidural metastases are breast, lung, and prostate pri-mary tumors. Recognition of spinal cord compression is critical for emergency management. High-dose intravenous cortico-steroids are administered empirically during the evaluation period. The appropriate diagnostic test is an immediate mag-netic resonance imaging (MRI) of the entire spine.

## Signs and Symptoms

Table 5-1 summarizes the signs and symptoms by location.

### Symptoms

- Pain is the first symptom in >90% of patients presenting with epidural metastasis and occurs less frequently with intradural tumors.
- Mechanisms of pain include spinal cord ischemia and traction on the periosteum, dura, nearby soft tissues, and nerve roots.

**Table 5-1**  Types of Spinal Cord Tumors by Location and Associated
Signs and Symptoms

|  | *Intramedullary* | *Intradural and Extramedullary* | *Epidural* |
|---|---|---|---|
| Symptoms | Pain + <br> Sensory loss <br> Early sphincter dysfunction | Pain, metastatic +++ <br> Pain, primary tumor + <br> Radicular or local <br> Sensory loss—radicular | Pain +++ <br> Radicular or local |
| Signs | Decreased rectal tone <br> Post-void residual <br> Sacral sparing <br> Spasticity <br> Upper motor neuron signs | Radicular or segmental weakness and sensory loss <br> Upper motor neuron signs | |
| Common tumors | Ependymoma <br> Astrocytoma | Meningioma | Metastatic |

- Pain occasionally can be absent in adults and more often is absent in children. If other neurologic symptoms suggestive of myelopathy are present, without pain, the clinician should evaluate for spinal cord tumor.
- Pain tends to begin as a local ache and is made worse by lying down, Valsalva manuever, and sometimes by twisting. Vertebral metastasis complicated by spinal instability is an exception to this, with pain being relieved by immobility.
- Spine pain that occurs at night and is eased when the patient is ambulatory more likely is due to tumor than a herniated disc. The latter tends to improve when the patient is lying down, especially on the side with the knees flexed.
- Sensory loss without pain or weakness is rare as a presentation for spinal cord compression.
- Patients with thoracic level spinal cord compression may experience a band-like sensation around the chest.
- Lhermitte's sign (extremity paresthesias precipitated by neck flexion) can occur with cervical spine lesions.
- Facial numbness can occur with high cervical (C2, C3) lesions.
- Changes in bowel and bladder habits, particularly urinary retention with overflow incontinence, usually occur late in the course of epidural spinal cord compression but are seen in a small percentage of patients at presentation.

## Signs

The patient should be examined for spinal tenderness or evidence of instability. If instability is suspected, the patient should be immobilized and a neurosurgical consultation requested. A detailed neurologic examination is an integral part of the evaluation of patients with suspected spinal cord involvement by tumor. The neurologic exam helps localize the lesion anatomically and may disclose other asymptomatic sites of tumor involvement. For example, an abnormality of the cranial nerves along with a myelopathy suggests multifocal tumor involvement or a more diffuse process such as leptomeningeal spread of tumor.

The motor examination may disclose radicular weakness (lower motor neuron) at the level of the lesion or a spastic paraparesis (upper motor neuron) below the level of the lesion. When present, sensory loss usually starts in the feet and rises proximally, mimicking the progression of a peripheral neuropathy, although the rate of progression is faster. Sacral sparing is considered typical of intramedullary lesions but is also seen in up to 20% of patients with spinal cord compression. Sensory loss with cauda equina compression generally is dermatomal and bilateral. The patient should be examined for evidence of urinary bladder retention by palpating the bladder and checking for post-void residual. Urinary retention usually is made worse by bedrest and narcotic analgesics. An indwelling bladder catheter often is needed to avoid acute retention, the associated discomfort, and overflow incontinence. Rectal sphincter tone may be normal, diminished, or absent. Constipation can occur and should be managed expectantly.

Deep tendon reflexes can be absent at the level of the lesion but usually are brisk below the level of the lesion. When spinal shock is present, reflexes are absent below the level of the lesion. Although Babinski signs commonly are present with spinal cord compression, normal plantar responses do not exclude the presence of spinal cord compression. After paralysis occurs, there often is no response to plantar stimulation acutely.

## Pearls and Caveats

- Both late and acute compression can manifest as motor flaccidity in affected muscle groups.
- The pattern of weakness is important to note. Cord compression primarily causes upper motor neuron weakness (legs weaker proximally).
- Fast-growing lesions, which usually are metastatic, do not localize as well in terms of signs and symptoms as slower-growing lesions.
- Cauda equina syndrome is a syndrome distinct from actual cord compression, in which lower motor neuron weakness in the legs (distal

**Table 5-2**  Differential Diagnosis of Spinal Cord Involvement in the Cancer Patient

| | |
|---|---|
| Tumor | Epidural compression by metastatic tumor |
| | Leptomeningeal metastasis—less common |
| | Intramedullary metastasis—rare |
| | Paraneoplastic myelopathy |
| Effects of treatments | Radiation myelopathy |
| | Myelopathy due to intrathecal chemotherapy |
| Infection | Epidural abscess |
| | Herpes (*Cytomegalovirus* or *Herpes simplex*) myelitis |
| | Fungal or tuberculous meningitis |
| Vascular | Epidural hematoma |
| | Vascular malformation |
| Degenerative | Herniated disc |
| | Vertebral collapse due to osteoporosis |

legs weaker than proximal) is accompanied by early sensory changes and sphincter dysfunction.

## Evaluation and Differential Diagnosis

Evaluation for suspected spinal cord involvement should be performed on an emergent basis if there is any evidence of neurologic compromise or radicular pain. Many patients with systemic cancer develop vertebral metastasis; only a subset develop epidural metastasis with neurologic compromise. Spinal cord symptoms in cancer patients also can be due to the effects of certain treatments, infections, and factors unrelated to the patient's tumor. Table 5-2 lists other important causes of spinal cord symptoms in the cancer patient.

## Suggested Reading

Posner JB. *Neurologic Complications of Cancer.* Philadelphia: F.A. Davis, 1995.
Schold SC Jr, Burger PC, Mendelsohn DB, et al. *Primary Tumors of the Brain and Spinal Cord.* Boston: Butterworth–Heinemann, 1997.

# 6

# Approach to
# the Evaluation
# of New Patients

The initial evaluation of a patient with a newly diagnosed tumor of the nervous system is a critical step toward appropriate management and patient care. The most important portions of the initial evaluation are a detailed history and a thorough examination. This process serves to identify the extent and nature of neurologic deficit, provides diagnostic clues, can help disclose a source of metastasis, or may identify a genetic process associated with a primary central nervous system (CNS) tumor. The history also may disclose recent symptoms that require urgent attention or chronic conditions that will affect the patient's management. Also important, the initial evaluation is the first opportunity to develop rapport with the patient. At some point following the initial evaluation, the clinician should be able to convey to the patient the nature of the condition. Here, we discuss the process of evaluating patients with newly diagnosed intracranial and spinal lesions and important initial diagnostic and therapeutic considerations.

## General Approach

A complete history and physical exam is performed with special attention to the areas of urgent concern to the patient or pressing medical conditions. Table 6-1 lists some important areas of investigation to be pursued during the initial evaluation of patients. Because these patients frequently have multiple, ongoing problems, a multidisciplinary team approach to the evaluation can be quite helpful. Inclusion on the team will depend on the specific situation and the areas may include neurology or neuro-oncology, neurosurgery, radiation oncology, medical oncology, ophthalmology, physical therapy, occupational therapy, nutrition, clinical pharmacy, and social work.

**Table 6-1**  Important Issues to Address During the Initial Assessment, Implications, and Management Strategies

| Clinical Problem | Implications | Management Strategies |
|---|---|---|
| Hemiparesis or paraplegia | Impaired mobility or self-care<br>Increased risk of DVT | Consider corticosteroids<br>Physical therapy<br>Occupational therapy |
| Speech impairment: | | |
| Aphasia | Localizes to dominant hemisphere<br>Presents communication barrier for caregivers | Speech therapy<br>Swallowing evaluation<br>Increase time needed with patient and caregiver for instructions |
| Dysarthria | Cortical, subcortical, brainstem or neuromuscular<br>May be associated with dysphagia → aspiration risk | Speech therapy<br>Swallowing evaluation |
| Seizures | Impairs quality of life<br>Recurrent seizures may increase ICP or worsen neurologic deficit<br>Risk of injury | Initiate anticonvulsant therapy, consult a neurologist<br>Discuss seizure precautions, educate patient and caregiver |
| Headaches | Impairs quality of life<br>May herald increased ICP<br>May herald hydrocephalus | Appropriate pain medication<br>Consider corticosteroids<br>Evaluate for increased ICP<br>Review for secondary causes |
| Visual deficits: | | |
| Decreased acuity or visual field loss | Impairs quality of life<br>May relate to specific etiology or localization<br>Impairs reading of instructions, prescriptions<br>Impairs mobility, increases risk of injury | Identify specific condition if possible<br>Enlist assistance of caregiver<br>Evaluation by ophthalmologist |

*continues*

**Table 6-1**  Important Issues to Address During the Initial Assessment, Implications, and Management Strategies  *continued*

| Clinical Problem | Implications | Management Strategies |
|---|---|---|
| Diplopia | May herald increased ICP<br>Decreases quality of life | Evaluate and treat for increased ICP<br>Alternating eye patches<br>Ophthalmology evaluation for prism glasses when stabilized |
| Nausea and vomiting | Possible increased ICP<br>May relate to treatments<br>Impairs quality of life | Symptomatic treatment<br>Evaluate for underlying causes |
| Symptoms of DVT or PE | Life threatening | Evaluate and treat |
| Medical conditions: | | |
| Diabetes | Impaired glucose tolerance<br>Affects use of corticosteroids<br>Increased risk of infections | Use corticosteroids cautiously<br>Monitor blood glucose closely, endocrinology consultation<br>Monitor for infections as appropriate |
| Cardiac disease | Impaired cardiac reserve | Restricts use of certain chemotherapy agents<br>Careful hydration for chemotherapy<br>Optimize medical treatment—cardiology consultation |
| Pulmonary disease or smoking history | Impaired pulmonary reserve<br>Increased risk of pulmonary infections | Restricts use of certain chemotherapy agents<br>Optimize medical management, pulmonary consultation |
| Financial barriers | May restrict options for therapy<br>May restrict hospice benefits | Arrange patient counseling regarding benefits and options |
| Geographical factors | Restricts access to subspecialty care<br>Restricts availability of emergency care | Maintain close contact with local physician<br>Patient education |
| Pre-existing patient biases and beliefs | Affects perception of disease process<br>Affects perception of value of treatment | Discuss and address patient concerns<br>Enlist support of family and other caregivers |

DVT, deep venous thrombosis; ICP, intracranial pressure; PE, pulmonary embolis.

## Intracranial Mass Lesions

When a CNS tumor is suspected based on the history or neurologic examination, cranial magnetic resonance imaging (MRI) with gadolinium enhancement usually is the diagnostic procedure of choice. MRI scanning best characterizes most primary brain tumors. Patients with metastasis are best imaged with MRI. Smaller lesions sometimes are missed on computed tomography (CT), and the presence of multiple lesions affects prognosis and management. CT scanning is chosen over MRI if the patient is unstable, hemorrhage is suspected, or MRI scanning is not immediately available. Tumor calcification also is seen more easily on CT. Table 9-2 lists the radiographic and clinical features of the more common primary and metastatic CNS tumors. Despite recent advances in neuroimaging, brain tumors occasionally can be mistaken for other conditions and vice versa.

## Spinal Lesions

The etiology of spinal cord lesions relates primarily to location (epidural, intramedullary). Suspected spinal cord compression is a neurologic emergency. MRI scanning is the diagnostic test of choice for evaluating suspected spinal cord tumors. Because spinal cord involvement often occurs at more than one level, the entire spine should be imaged.

## Synthesis

A tissue diagnosis always should be considered in cases of newly diagnosed intracranial mass lesions. When there is no history of cancer, a careful history and physical examination are sufficient evaluations prior to obtaining a tissue diagnosis. Table 6-2 lists some well-defined situations that may obviate the need for a tissue diagnosis. Such a decision should be reached only in conjunction with physicians experienced in the specific tumor under consideration. For example, decisions about surgical accessibility should be made by a neurosurgeon experienced in tumor surgery. Because sampling error is a significant issue in the evaluation of brain tumors, radiographic and clinical correlations are critical. For example, a tumor may be biopsied peripherally, providing a misleading lower-grade pathology than actually is present. Accurate diagnosis of a CNS neoplasm is critical in designing optimal therapy and providing appropriate counseling for the patient and family. Furthermore, the available therapies for CNS tumors can be substantially toxic and even fatal. A multidisciplinary conference, such as a tumor board, provides an optimal platform for discussion of newly diagnosed patients.

**Table 6-2** Tumors That May Not Require Tissue Diagnosis

| | |
|---|---|
| Known systemic malignancy | The most common cause of an intracranial mass lesion in patients with known malignancy is brain metastasis. |
| | In certain circumstances, surgery is therapeutic or necessary to distinguish metastasis from other processes and thus guide appropriate therapy. |
| Pontine gliomas | Appearance of an enlarged pons without exophytic component is characteristic. |
| | Risks of biopsy outweigh risks of empiric therapy. |
| Marker-positive tumors: Endodermal sinus tumor, alpha fetoprotein Choriocarcinoma, beta sub-unit of human chorionic gonadotropin | Germ cell tumors that secrete characteristic proteins detected in the CSF sometimes can be diagnosed with the combination of a characteristic MRI and CSF examination. A histologic diagnosis is needed if markers are elevated only modestly. |
| Optic nerve, chiasm, and optic nerve sheath tumors | Carefully consider risks (impairment of vision) vs. benefits (improvement of vision) due to surgery and risks of empiric therapy vs. benefit of tissue diagnosis. |

CSF, cerebrospinal fluid; MRI, magnetic resonance imaging.

# 7

# Practical Strategies for Providing Appropriate Patient Care

There is no question that the clinical management of neuro-oncology patients is challenging. Complex medical problems, social situations, and frequently poor prognosis can make the care of these patients time consuming, frustrating, and emotionally demanding. Furthermore, under current reimbursement programs, clinicians often are ill compensated financially for their efforts. However, if we are to help individual patients and ultimately make advances in treating these tumors, meticulous and compassionate care of patients with neurologic malignancies are critical.

Approaching the care of these patients is different from caring for patients with acute problems or illnesses of short duration. All cancer patients are confronted with a continuing and ongoing series of challenges; and for brain tumor patients, these challenges are especially formidable. In turn, their physicians and other caregivers are faced with the chronic care of patients with multiple ongoing medical and social needs. Both patient and physician benefit from an approach that recognizes and foresees these demands. A comprehensive multidisciplinary approach that anticipates and responds to ongoing patient needs is the way to provide optimal care for these patients. Appendix 1 lists agencies and organizations that may be useful in determining treatment options and offering social services and other support.

## Challenges

Tumors affecting the central nervous system (CNS) can alter a patient's cognitive and intellectual functioning, mobility, and may cause disabling pain. These factors can profoundly influence patient management. Brain tumor patients may demonstrate any or all of the following problems, which are not always related to tumor location or size. Also, some of these problems can relate to previous or ongoing antitumor therapies. Recognition of these problems is important for optimal patient management planning. It is equally important not to assume, in individual patients, that all these deficits are present.

- Patients may have *poor insight* regarding their own level of function and therefore may overestimate their ability to be independent, follow instructions, manage medications, and drive.
- Concomitant *stress or depression* may cause patients to underrate their own abilities, causing inappropriate burdens for caregivers.
- *Memory problems* may lead to noncompliance with instructions and medications as well as inaccurate reporting of symptoms.
- Subtle *language problems* may interfere with comprehension of verbal and written instructions.
- Patients may have *psychomotor retardation*, making them unable to perform certain activities due to poor initiation.
- *Visual-spatial difficulties* may cause difficulty with directions (patients get lost in hospital corridors).
- *Behavior and personality changes* cause difficulties in interpersonal relationships, both with family members and professional caregivers.
- *Poor attention span* and ability to recall information can result in a poor understanding of the tumor and treatment issues. This may prolong clinic visits or prompt multiple subsequent phone calls.

These problems present significant challenges regarding patient management, compliance, ability to provide informed consent, interpersonal relationships, and quality of life. The ability to drive safely and live independently are major issues and areas of potential conflict between clinicians, their patients, and members of the patient's support system.

## Management Strategies

- *Give instructions both orally and in written form* for the patient to take home. This assists patients in maintaining some responsibility for their own care, yet provides a written reference for others to use. Repetition and rephrasing is important for many patients.
- *Use a consistent format* of written instructions, so that a patient can expect where to find information on the page.

- *Write down new or important diagnoses* for the patient or family to refer to at home.
- *Identify one reliable caregiver* to serve as a contact point. This caregiver should be present during encounters with the patient and should communicate with all others involved with the patient's care. Avoid independent communication with multiple caregivers to limit confusion.
- *Pictures and diagrams* are helpful, particularly if a patient has a language deficit.
- *A team approach,* using clinicians with different areas of expertise, is helpful.
- *Provide a reliable and simple method for the patient to seek help.* It is not reasonable to expect a brain tumor patient to navigate through complicated phone mail instructions or caregivers who are unfamiliar with the patient's situation to solicit help.
- *Minimize sedating drug use* whenever possible.
- *Establish a nonthreatening method of monitoring medication usage.* The use of a daily "pill box" can be very helpful. Patients can remain responsible for taking their own medications, while the caregiver has a method of verifying that medications are taken accurately. Counting pills in the bottle and correlating with dates prescriptions were dispensed are other ways of monitoring medication use.
- *Establish a method of monitoring PRN medications* so that the patient does not inadvertently overdose medications, especially narcotics, and the caregiver has an indication of symptom frequency such as headaches. Often, patients will take more narcotics than they realize and yet omit the history of headaches unless specifically asked.

# 8

# Introduction to Clinical Trials

The National Cancer Institute defines a *clinical trial* as a "test [of] new treatments in people with cancer. . . . Clinical trials test many types of treatment such as new drugs, new approaches to surgery or radiation therapy, new combinations of treatments, or new methods such as gene therapy."

Clinical trials are our link to medical progress. Through clinical trials we gain knowledge that will benefit patients in the future. For brain tumor patients, clinical trials may provide improved survival and enhanced quality of life over what might be expected with conventional therapy.

Although participation in a clinical trial can be beneficial, it also presents medical, logistical, ethical, psychosocial, and financial challenges to the patient and care providers. Physicians and patients should carefully consider such issues before deciding to participate in a clinical trial. The National Cancer Institute's guidebook, *Taking Part in Clinical Trials: What Cancer Patients Need to Know*, is an excellent reference for patients who are considering participation in a clinical trial. This guide explains clinical trials in lay language and can be ordered free of charge from the National Cancer Institute (NCI/Novartis Oncology, NIH Publication No. 98-4270, 1998). To order this booklet, contact the NCI:

Phone: 1-800-4-CANCER
Fax: 301-402-5874
E-mail: cancermail@cips.nci.nih.gov
Website: http://www.nci.nih.gov
Address: National Cancer Institute, National Institutes of Health,
    Rockville, MD 20852

- Treating physicians need to assess the patient's understanding of the study and his or her willingness to comply with the treatment and monitoring schedule.
- Physicians can assist patients by helping to interpret the potential benefits and risks of a clinical trial, as well as the eligibility and exclusion criteria.

- Many patients have pre-existing biases about treatment options including participation in clinical trials. It is the physician's responsibility to address such biases as appropriate and to assist the patient in making a decision.
- Although every patient should have the opportunity to consider participation in a clinical trial, not all patients are candidates. The specific study protocol will list eligibility and exclusion criteria.
- Most clinical trials for systemic tumors exclude patients with brain metastases. However, such patients may be eligible for studies focused on treatment of metastatic tumor to the brain. These studies often are quite specific about criteria such as number of metastatic sites, tumor size, and previous treatment.
- Over the past few years, it has become easier for patients to participate in clinical trials without having to travel long distances. The creation of CCOPs (community clinical oncology programs) and CGOPs (cooperative group outreach programs) has allowed community-based oncologists to enter patients on many national clinical trials and receive shipments of the investigational drugs often used to treat patients on these trials. However, in communities without an oncologist, patients need to travel to undergo evaluation and treatment. Management of adverse effects, as well as routine monitoring between treatments, often can be done by primary care physician through communication with the study physician.
- To receive care from a specialized brain tumor center, many patients must travel to a medical center in another city, take up residence in that city during and immediately after treatment, and occasionally relocate for weeks or months at a time. It is important to discuss and clarify the logistical details of such a decision before treatment begins. Some patients may be physically or emotionally unable to travel whereas others welcome and seek out such opportunities. Physicians can help by guiding patients to information sources about the community in which they will receive treatment. Research-oriented medical centers often have staff responsible for assisting with housing, transportation, and other needs, as well as for providing liaison services to primary care providers.

## Types of Clinical Trials

It is important for physicians and patients to understand the types of clinical trials available.

### Phase I Trials

- Phase I trials are designed to determine the maximum tolerated dose and dose-limiting side effects of new agents. Such an agent, which is not yet approved for human use by the Food and Drug Administration, is termed an *investigational new drug* (IND).

- Alternative routes of administration of FDA approved drugs are initially investigated in phase I trials.
- Phase I trials may be appealing to some brain tumor patients but, in general, are reserved for those who have exhausted other, more conventional options.
- Some patients, or their physicians, may be sufficiently concerned about the risks of such studies and decline participation.

## Phase II Trials

- Phase II trials are preliminary efficacy studies and endpoints typically include response rate, time to progression, and the incidence of toxicities.
- Either INDs or novel combinations or schedules of FDA-approved drugs are studied in this manner.
- Phase II trials typically target a specific patient population with a specific tumor type and stage. In general, phase II studies for brain tumors are available to patients with tumor recurrence following standard therapy.

## Phase III Trials

- Phase III trials compare new therapies to "standard therapy." Patients are randomized to one or more treatment "arms," which dictate the treatment they receive. Endpoints typically include response rate, survival, and toxicity.
- Randomization is unacceptable to some patients; an open discussion of the concept of randomization is important for patients considering participation in a randomized trial.
- In general, phase III trials are offered to patients with newly diagnosed brain tumors.

## Institutional Review Boards

Clinical trials are submitted for approval to each participating institution's Review Board, whose task is to monitor clinical research to ensure that scientific and ethical standards are met. These committees review the informed consent documents that patients sign before starting research-based treatment.

## Informed Consent

The process of informed consent includes (1) verbal discussion between the patient and physician regarding the nature of the study and anticipated risks and benefits, (2) reading and signing the consent form, and (3) supplying the patient with a copy of the consent form for his or her records.

If possible, patients should be given the opportunity to take the consent form home to read it before signing it. The physician can perform a valuable service by acting as the patient's advocate, reading the consent form and discussing it to ensure that it is understood.

## Financial Considerations

Financial aspects of clinical trials vary. Some studies include funding for all components of care, including medications, laboratory testing, and hospitalization, while the patient is a participant. More commonly, studies pay only for selected expenses, such as investigational drugs or tests done solely for research purposes. Some include no financial assistance at all. It is important that the patient or person responsible for the patient's finances understands the financial ramifications of a clinical trial under consideration. This information often is provided via the informed consent document or through other, supplemental written guidelines.

## Finding Out about Available Clinical Trials

Some patients already will have consulted one or more of the organizations listed in the Resources section listed at the back of the National Cancer Institute's guide; others will be unaware of the option of participating in a clinical trial. Treatment options, including clinical trials, should be discussed with patients as part of good medical care, so that patients are aware of their options. Groups such as the American Brain Tumor Association, Brain Tumor Foundation of Canada, and National Brain Tumor Society can provide listings of clinical research opportunities. The National Cancer Institute and American Cancer Society also can focus on clinical trials specifically for primary brain tumor patients or for patients with brain metastases from other primary tumors.

## Suggested Reading

Friedman MA. Clinical trials. In GP Murphy, W Lawrence, RE Lenhard (eds). *American Cancer Society Textbook of Clinical Oncology.* Atlanta: American Cancer Society, 1995:194–197.

Livingston RB, Carter SK. Experimental design and clinical trials: Clinical perspective. In SK Carter, E Glatstein, RB Livingston (eds). *Principles of Cancer Treatment.* New York: McGraw-Hill, 1982:34–45.

# III

## Diagnostic Procedures

# 9

# Diagnostic Imaging of the Brain and Spinal Cord

Modern diagnostic imaging has advanced our understanding of and ability to diagnose brain and spinal cord tumors and neurologic complications of systemic cancer. The imaging studies commonly used in neuro-oncology are computed tomography (CT) and magnetic resonance imaging (MRI). Less commonly used are myelography, positron emission tomography (PET), and diagnostic angiography. Magnetic resonance spectroscopy (MRS) is an emerging technique that may prove valuable in following treated patients. Neuro-imaging is an essential portion of the initial evaluation of neurologic symptoms and for following the patient for response or complications. Although MRI is more costly than CT, it is the preferred imaging modality in most situations. Both CT and MRI can be performed with IV contrast agents that "enhance" areas of blood-brain barrier breakdown. In some classes of tumors, such as the astrocytomas, the extent of such enhancement correlates with the degree of malignancy. However, some benign tumors enhance vividly, including meningiomas, pituitary adenomas, and pilocytic astrocytomas. Review of confusing or complicated cases with a neuroradiologist can be very valuable.

Table 9-1 lists the relative advantages and disadvantages of CT and MRI scanning in neuro-oncology. Although MRI scans are superior to CT for most neuro-oncology evaluations, CT plays a valuable role in excluding hemorrhage, is easier to perform on unstable patients, and usually is more rapidly

**Table 9-1**    Comparison of CT and MRI Scanning of Brain and Spinal Tumors

|     | Advantages | Disadvantages |
| --- | --- | --- |
| CT | Rapid<br>Identifies calcification in tumor<br>Identifies hemorrhage<br>Patient movement degrades images<br>less than for MRI | Lower resolution<br>Poor visualization of posterior fossa<br>and spinal cord<br>IV contrast allergy<br>Seizures following contrast in some<br>patients with brain tumors |
| MRI | Higher resolution<br>Better images of posterior fossa<br>Best images of spine | Requires cooperative patient<br>Patient movement degrades image<br>quality<br>Claustrophobia may prevent opti-<br>mal examination<br>More costly |

available. CT also is superior for evaluation of tumors with regard to possible bone involvement and proximity to bony structures. Despite the significant advances in neuro-imaging over the past decade, radiographic characteristics can be nonspecific and tissue confirmation is essential in most patients.

A detailed description of the methods and physics pertinent to neuro-imaging can be found in standard neuro-radiology texts (such as that listed in the Suggested Reading). Table 9-2 lists important diagnostic features in neuro-imaging of tumors and related processes. The presence of hemorrhage is of some diagnostic value. Table 9-3 lists primary and metastatic tumors that have a tendency to bleed. Blood is bright on unenhanced CT scans. Table 9-4 describes the signal characteristics of blood on MRI, based on the chronology of the hemorrhage. Intracranial calcification is associated with some tumors but also occurs in specific areas as a normal finding, as shown in Table 9-5. Table 9-6 lists the intracranial tumors characteristically associated with a cystic component.

**Table 9-2** Differential Diagnosis of Intracranial Lesions by Radiographic Features

| Tumor or Process | Single or Multiple[a] | Radiographic Features and Comments |
|---|---|---|
| **Fibrillary Astrocytomas** | | |
| Glioblastoma | Single | CT: Low-density mass, + enhancement, usually heterogeneous or ring enhancing, significant mass effect<br>MRI: Hypointense on T1, hyperintense on T2, significant mass effect, ++ enhancement |
| Anaplastic astrocytoma | Single | CT: Low-density mass, +/– enhancement<br>MRI: Iso- or hypointense on T1, increased T2 signal, some mass effect, +/– enhancement |
| Low-grade astrocytoma | Single | CT: Low-density mass, no enhancement<br>MRI: Iso- or hypointense on T1, hyperintense on T2, minimal mass effect, no enhancement |
| **Oligodendroglioma** | | |
| Anaplastic | Single | CT: Hypodense, +/– enhancement, heterogeneous or ring, sometimes calcified<br>MRI: Hypo- or isointense on T1, hyperintense T2, +/– enhancement |
| Low grade | Single | CT: Low-density mass, minimal enhancement, calcified<br>MRI: Iso- or hypointense on T1, hyperintense on T2, minimal enhancement |
| **Ependymoma** | Single | CT: Isodense, calcified (50%), cystic<br>MRI: Heterogeneous signal, + enhancement<br>Fourth ventricle, supratentorial |
| **Meningiomas** | | |
| Typical | Single, occasionally multiple | CT: Dura-based mass, hyper- or isodense, homogenous, and +++ enhancement<br>MRI: Dura-based mass, hyper- or isointense on T1, +/– surrounding increased signal on T2<br>Homogenous +++ enhancement |
| Atypical | Single, occasionally multiple | Same as preceding except irregular margins and shape as tumor grows along dura at base of skull |

*continues*

**Table 9-2**   Differential Diagnosis of Intracranial Lesions by Radiographic
Features   *continued*

| Tumor or Process | Single or Multiple[a] | Radiographic Features and Comments |
|---|---|---|
| Anaplastic, malignant | Single, occasionally multiple | Dura-based mass, may invade brain, irregular margins, and extensive brain edema<br>Cannot reliably distinguish malignant from benign meningioma radiographically |
| **Medulloblastoma** | Single | CT: Hyperdense, enhancement +++ and homogenous<br>MRI: Iso- or hypointense on T1, hyperintense on T2, enhancement usually vivid and homogenous but may be absent (especially after treatment and in older patients)<br>CSF spread common (leptomeningeal disease)<br>Cysts, hemorrhage, and calcification common<br>Midline cerebellum (85%, children)<br>Lateral cerebellum (15%, young adults) |
| **Other PNETs** | | CT: hyperdense, heterogeneous enhancement (sometimes minimal)<br>MRI: heterogeneous signal<br>Cysts, hemorrhage, and calcification are common<br>CSF spread common (leptomeningeal disease) |
| **PCNSL** | | |
| Non-HIV | Single or multiple | CT: Iso- or hyperdense, enhance homogeneously<br>MRI: Iso- or hyperdense on T1, hyperdense on T2, enhance homogeneously<br>MRI better to detect leptomeningeal involvement |
| HIV | Single or multiple | CT: Central necrosis with ring, +/− enhancement<br>MRI: Iso- or hyperdense on T1, hyperdense on T2, ring enhancement or no enhancement<br>MRI better to detect leptomeningeal involvement |

*continues*

**Table 9-2** Differential Diagnosis of Intracranial Lesions by Radiographic Features *continued*

| Tumor or Process | Single or Multiple[a] | Radiographic Features and Comments |
|---|---|---|
| **Metastasis** | | |
| Brain metastasis | 50% single, 50% multiple | Solid or ring enhancing, peritumoral edema, locate at gray/white junction, pineal, pituitary, choroid plexus |
| Dural metastasis | Single | May mimic meningioma<br>Usually from breast, lung, prostate, or systemic lymphoma<br>Edema in underlying brain |
| **Brain abscess** | Single or multiple | Ring or solid enhancement, locate at gray/white junction, signs of sepsis (fever, chills, increased white blood count) usually absent |
| **Vascular** | | |
| Hemorrhage | | Acute: Blood is increased on T1 signal on MRI and bright on unenhanced CT scan for all types of hemorrhage |
| Epidural | | Crescent-shaped blood collection |
| Subdural | | Convex blood collection, history of multiple falls |
| Subarachnoid | | Blood in subarachnoid spaces |
| Embolus | Single, occasionally multiple | Marantic endocarditis<br>Tumor embolus |
| Venous sinus thrombosis | | Can see single or multiple venous infarcts, which may be hemorrhagic<br>Consider hypercoagulable states |
| Stroke | Single, occasionally multiple | Findings depend on stage of ischemia<br>In general hypodense (on CT) or hyperintense (on MRI) and some mass effect<br>Abnormality wedge shaped and in a vascular distribution<br>+/– cortical enhancement |
| Malformations | Single, rarely multiple | Heterogeneous masses, sometimes with evidence of hemorrhage<br>Rarely can harbor metastasis |

*continues*

**Table 9-2**  Differential Diagnosis of Intracranial Lesions by Radiographic Features *continued*

| Tumor or Process | Single or Multiple[a] | Radiographic Features and Comments |
|---|---|---|
| **Radiation necrosis** | Single, rarely multiple | Ring or inhomogeneous enhancement, mass effect<br>Cannot distinguish from tumor radiographically |
| **Radiation leuko-encephalopathy** | Single or multiple | Areas of increased signal in white matter on T2 images, which can become confluent |
| **Multiple sclerosis** | Multiple, occasionally single | MS plaques generally increased on T2, may have surrounding ring enhancement and mild mass effect<br>Seek history of prior transient CNS symptoms or optic neuritis |
| **Status epilepticus** | Single | Can induce area of increased T2 signal, sometimes enhances, minimal mass effect, usually temporal lobes |
| **Progressive multifocal leukoencephalopathy** | Multiple | Multiple areas of periventricular involvement with little or no mass effect<br>Increased signal on T2 MRI, hypo- or isodense to brain on T1 MRI, rarely enhancement<br>Occurs in immunosuppressed patients |
| **Old trauma** | | Area(s) of increased T2 signal, negative mass effect, no enhancement, tip of temporal or frontal lobes<br>Seek history |
| **Surgical changes** | | Meningeal enhancement, enhancement of operative bed, fat packing visualized as increased on T1 |

PNET, primitive neuroectodermal tumor; PCNSL, primary CNS lymphoma.
[a]Some single lesions can be mistaken for multiple lesions.

**Table 9-3**  Hemorrhage within CNS Tumors

| Primary Tumors | Metastatic Tumors |
|---|---|
| Glioblastoma | Choriocarcinoma |
| Oligodendroglioma | Thyroid |
| PNETs | Melanoma |
| | Lung |
| | Renal |

PNET, primitive neuroectodermal tumor.

**Table 9-4**   MRI Signal Characteristics of Hemorrhage

| Blood Product | Timing after Bleeding | Corresponding MRI Signal Abnormality |
|---|---|---|
| Oxyhemoglobin | 12 hours | Isointense on T1 and T2 |
| Deoxyhemoglobin | 1–7 days | Isointense on T1<br>Hypointense on T2 |
| Methemoglobin | 5 days to months (sometimes years) | Hyperintense on T1<br>Hypointense on T2 (if intracellular)<br>Hyperintense on T2 (if extracellular) |
| Hemosiderin | Weeks to years | Isointense to slightly hypointense on T1<br>Hypointense on T2<br>Very hypointense on gradient echo scans |

**Table 9-5**   Calcification of Tumors, Infections, and Normal Structures

| Tumor or Process (% calcification) | Location and Comments |
|---|---|
| **Oligodendroglioma (50%)** | Cerebral hemispheres, white matter |
| **Astrocytoma (7–10%)** | Cerebral hemispheres, white matter |
| **Ependymoma**<br>  Infratentorial (40–60%)<br>  Supratentorial (30%) | Cerebellum, brain stem, supratentorial |
| **Ganglion cell tumors (40–50%)** | Temporal lobes |
| **Dermoid tumor (>90%)** | Cerebellar-pontine angle |
| **Teratoma (>90%)** | |
| **Epidermoid tumor (rare)** | |
| **Untreated metastasis, pituitary adenoma, lipoma, epidermoid, medulloblastoma** | Calcification is rare |
| **Meningioma (10–20%)** | Convexities, base of skull, spine |
| **Craniopharyngioma**<br>  Calcification common in children (70–80%)<br>  Frequency of calcification decreases with age at diagnosis | Suprasellar, intrasellar, or both |
| **Vascular malformations**<br>  Cavernous angiomas (50%)<br>  Arteriovenous malformations (25%)<br>  Aneurysms (5%) | |
| **Chronic infections**<br>  Toxoplasmosis<br>  Cytomegalovirus<br>  Tuberculosis<br>  Cysticercosis | |

*continues*

**Table 9-5**   Calcification of Tumors, Infections, and Normal Structures
*continued*

| Tumor or Process (% calcification) | Location and Comments |
|---|---|
| **Normal structures**<br>Prevalence of calcification increases with age<br>Calcification in children under 9 years, suspect neoplasia | Pineal gland (rare in children under 9)<br>Choroid plexus (rare in children under 9) involves lateral ventricles, rare in third or fourth ventricle<br>Falx<br>Tentorium (less common than falx)<br>Arachnoid granulations: appear as round calcified structures, parasagittal<br>Dural plaques<br>Basal ganglia (usually idiopathic)<br>Blood vessels |

**Table 9-6**   Tumors Commonly Associated with a Cystic Component

Pilocytic astrocytomas

Ganglion cell tumors

PNET

Ependymoma

Hemangioblastoma

Pleomorphic xanthoastrocytoma

Craniopharyngeoma

PNET, primitive neuroectodermal tumor.

## Pearls and Caveats in the Imaging of Brain Tumors and Central Nervous System Involvement of Cancer

- Postoperative scans to document the degree of resection should be obtained within 48 hours of surgery to avoid confusion with the expected postoperative enhancement that develops beyond this period and does not indicate residual tumor.
- Comparison of radiographic findings between MRI and CT scans is not always valid. In general, MRI is more sensitive to contrast enhancement than is CT.
- The degree of contrast enhancement does not always correlate with the degree of malignancy.

- Up to 40% of nonenhancing gliomas have anaplastic features histologically.
- Although melanoma, choriocarcinoma, and thyroid metastasis frequently are hemorrhagic, hemorrhagic brain metastases more often are due to lung cancer, because it is a more common source of metastasis.
- Because blood is hyperdense on CT and hyperintense on T1 MRI scans, the precontrast scans always should be reviewed to exclude the presence of blood as the cause of apparent enhancement.
- The radiologic findings of leptomeningeal tumor include diffuse or patchy leptomeningeal enhancement. However, a normal MRI does not exclude leptomeningeal tumor.
- Low-pressure syndromes that can follow lumbar puncture have been confused radiologically with leptomeningeal tumor.

## Pearls and Caveats in the Imaging of Spinal Cord Tumors

- Lesions may be several levels above the level based on the signs and symptoms.
- The entire spine should be imaged because metastatic disease to the spine often is multifocal and some primary spine tumors can be multifocal, such as ependymomas.
- Intradural tumor is visualized best on postgadolinium images, whereas epidural tumor is best visualized on unenhanced images.
- Vertebral compression fractures may harbor tumor metastasis.

## Suggested Reading

Osborn AG. *Diagnostic Neuroradiology.* St. Louis: Mosby, 1994.

# 10

# Lumbar Puncture and Cerebrospinal Fluid Analysis

Lumbar puncture (LP) and cerebrospinal fluid (CSF) analysis are important for the evaluation of some primary brain tumors, metastatic conditions, and neurologic complications of cancer. In general, patients with primary brain tumor or systemic cancer are at increased risk for complications of lumbar puncture. The risks of performing a lumbar puncture should be carefully evaluated prior to performing the procedure. The technique of lumbar puncture, normal CSF findings, and CSF findings in disease states are discussed here.

## Lumbar Puncture

### Evaluation Prior to Lumbar Puncture: Risks vs. Benefits

LP and CSF analysis can provide important diagnostic information and may be the only test that can establish diagnoses such as infectious meningitis. However, it is unsafe under certain circumstances, such as spinal block or a posterior fossa mass. The conditions for which LP is important or dangerous are summarized in Table 10-1. Neurologic consultation should be sought in cases of uncertainty about the safety of LP.

Contraindications to LP include

- In general, neuro-oncology patients with signs and symptoms of increased intracranial pressure (ICP) should *not* undergo lumbar puncture unless the presence of a mass lesion has been excluded by neuro-imaging. LP should not be performed on patients with brain lesions

**Table 10-1** Diagnostic Utility of Lumbar Puncture

| *Diseases for Which LP Is Not Helpful or Poses Significant Risks* | *Diseases for Which LP Is Helpful* |
|---|---|
| Brain metastasis | Leptomeningeal metastasis |
| Epidural spinal cord metastasis | Meningeal infections: |
| Brain abscess |   Bacterial meningitis |
| |   Tuberculous meningitis |
| Subdural hematoma |   Fungal meningitis |
| Ischemic stroke |   Viral meningitis |
| Embolic stroke |   CNS syphilis |
| | Subarachnoid hemorrhage |
| | Acute inflammatory demyelinating poly-neuropathy (Guillain-Barré syndrome) and chronic neuropathies |
| | CNS vasculitis |
| | Neurologic paraneoplastic syndromes |

CNS, central nervous system.

associated with mass effect, particularly of the temporal lobe or posterior fossa, because of the risk of cerebral herniation. LP in patients with large lesions also should be regarded with caution, even in the absence of mass effect.

- Papilledema is a relative contraindication to LP. Obtain a contrast-enhanced computed tomography (CT) or magnetic resonance imaging (MRI) scan to exclude focal lesions. If no intracranial mass is present, such a patient could undergo LP for diagnostic and possibly therapeutic purposes.
- Avoid LP in patients with a spinal cord block due to a mass lesion in the spinal cord at any level.
- Avoid LP in patients with an infection of the overlying skin or soft tissues.
- Be careful in patients with therapeutic anticoagulation or bleeding disorders:
  - Cancer patients should be evaluated with a complete blood count and clotting study prior to lumbar puncture.
  - Coumadin should be stopped for 3–4 days prior to lumbar puncture and the prothrombin time checked prior to the LP.
  - Heparin should be stopped for 1–2 hours before lumbar puncture and resumed no sooner than 2 hours after lumbar puncture is completed.

- Enoxaparin should be stopped 10 hours before lumbar puncture and resumed 2 hours after lumbar puncture is completed.
• Be careful in patients with thrombocytopenia or platelet dysfunction. Platelet transfusion should be given for patients undergoing LP who have platelet counts <20,000/mm$^3$ or suspected platelet dysfunction. The transfusion should be administered during, not prior to, the procedure. Only an experienced individual should perform an LP on any patient with a platelet count <50,000/mm$^3$. The smallest gauge needle is used and the procedure aborted after two unsuccessful passes.

## Lumbar Puncture Technique

Detailed information regarding the procedure can be found in the texts listed under Suggested Reading. Patients should be counseled carefully prior to the procedure to address their concerns, allay their fears, and obtain informed consent. Premedication with a benzodiazepine can be helpful in particularly anxious patients. Children usually require monitored sedation.

The procedure is best performed in the lateral decubitus position with the neuro-axis parallel to the floor. Deviation from this position causes an erroneously elevated opening pressure, although the sitting position occasionally is necessary for larger patients. Proper positioning is key to a successful procedure. The L4–L5 interspace is used most commonly, although the L3–L4 and L5–S1 spaces can be used as well. The opening pressure should be recorded with a manometer as soon as possible after successful placement of the needle in the subarachnoid space. Following this, CSF is collected, the stylet is replaced, and the needle is withdrawn. There is no evidence that bedrest following LP prevents any of the complications of LP; specifically, bedrest does not prevent post-LP headaches. Tests should be ordered based on the suspected condition and differential diagnosis. The CSF should be taken to the laboratory and processed immediately.

## Complications of Lumbar Puncture

• Cerebral herniation can occur up to 24 hours following LP. Any neurologic deterioration following LP should be carefully evaluated and a neurologist or neurosurgeon consulted. The treatment of cerebral herniation is covered in Chapter 43.
• Post-LP headaches occur in 5–25% of patients, more often in women than men. Smaller-gauge spinal needles are associated with fewer headaches, as is fewer passes of the spinal needle. Treatment is discussed in Chapter 41.
• Subdural hematoma and hygroma.

- Diplopia.
- Tinnitus.
- Spinal epidural or subdural hematoma.

## Cerebrospinal Fluid Composition and Pressure

### Normal Findings

Table 10-2 lists the normal laboratory values for CSF obtained at the lumbar level.

**Table 10-2**  CSF Findings for Routine Studies in Adults for Normal and Disease States

|  | *Normal Value* | *Disease States with Increase in Value* | *Disease States with Decrease in Value* |
|---|---|---|---|
| Opening pressure[a] | 65–200 mm CSF | Increased ICP:<br>  Mass lesion<br>  Meningitis<br>  Benign intracranial<br>    hypertension | Intracranial hypotension:<br>  Postlumbar puncture<br>  Spontaneous or trau-<br>    matic<br>  Spinal block |
| WBC (per mm$^3$) | <5 | Mild, 6–50:<br>  Leptomeningeal tumor<br>  Viral meningitis<br>  Cysticercosis<br>  CNS sarcoidosis<br>Moderate, 50–200:<br>  Tuberculous meningitis<br>  Cryptococcal meningitis<br>Marked, >200:<br>  Bacterial meningitis<br>  Syphilitic meningitis | Not applicable |
| RBC (per mm$^3$) | <5 | Subarachnoid hemorrhage<br>Herpes encephalitis<br>Traumatic lumbar puncture | Not applicable |
| Protein (mg/dl) | 20–45 | Slight increase, 45–75:<br>  Clearly abnormal but<br>    nonspecific finding in<br>    many CNS processes<br>  Viral meningitis or<br>    encephalitis<br>  HIV meningitis<br>Moderate increase, 75–100:<br>  Leptomeningeal tumor<br>  (may be normal) | Abnormally low, <20:<br>  Benign intracranial<br>    hypertension<br>  Recent large volume CSF<br>    removal by LP<br>  CSF leak<br>  Acute water intoxication<br>  Normal children <2 years |

*continues*

**Table 10-2**   CSF Findings for Routine Studies in Adults for Normal
and Disease States   *continued*

| | *Normal Value* | *Disease States with Increase in Value* | *Disease States with Decrease in Value* |
|---|---|---|---|
| | | Previous intrathecal chemotherapy | |
| | | Meningeal sarcoidosis | |
| | | Great increase, 100–500: | |
| | |   Bacterial, tuberculous, cryptococcal, syphilitic, cysticercosis meningitis | |
| | | Myxedema | |
| | | Neurofibroma in spinal cord | |
| | | Diabetic polyneuropathy | |
| | | Very great increase, 500–3600: | |
| | |   Purulent meningitis | |
| | |   Spinal block due to tumor or infection | |
| | |   Subarachnoid hemorrhage | |
| Glucose (mg/dl) | 45–80 (65% of blood glucose)[b] | = Hyperglycorrhachia<br>No diagnostic significance<br>Reflects hyperglycemia | = Hypoglycorrhachia<br>Low, 20–45:<br>  Meningitis: fungal, tuberculous, purulent, amebic, cysticercosis, trichinosis, syphilitic (rare), viral (mumps, herpes, CMV)<br>  Chemical meningitis following intrathecal chemotherapy<br>  Subarachnoid hemorrhage<br>  Hypoglycemia<br>  Meningeal sarcoidosis<br>  Leptomeningeal tumor<br>Markedly low, <20 (glucose is usually due to):<br>  Purulent meningitis<br>  Leptomeningeal tumor<br>  Tuberculosis |

WBC, white blood cell; RBC, red blood cell; CNS, central nervous system; CMV, cytomegalovirus.

[a]Patient in lateral decubitus position with spinal axis parallel to the floor. Obese patients may have normal pressures up to 250 mm $H_2O$.

[b]Hyperglycemia can mask a low CSF glucose. Obtain a simultaneous blood glucose for comparison.

- Protein concentration normally is lower in CSF obtained from an Ommaya (ventricular) reservoir or cisternal puncture than in CSF obtained from the lumbar site.
- Blood in the CSF due to a traumatic LP raises the CSF white blood cell (WBC) count proportional to the cell counts in blood. If the cell count and protein are measured from the same tube of CSF, the following guidelines are helpful to correct for the presence of blood:
  - Assuming normal peripheral complete blood count (CBC), subtract 1 WBC/mm$^3$ from the measured CSF WBC count for every 700 red blood cells (RBCs)/mm$^3$.
  - In the presence of anemia or leukocytosis,

    $$\text{Corrected CSF WBC count (mm}^3) = \frac{[\text{WBC}(f) - \text{WBC}(b)] \times \text{RBC}(f)}{\text{RBC}(b)}$$

    where
    WBC($f$) = measured WBC in bloody CSF/mm$^3$,
    WBC($b$) = measured WBC in peripheral blood/mm$^3$,
    RBC($f$)  = measured RBC in CSF/mm$^3$,
    RBC($b$) = measured RBC in peripheral blood/mm$^3$.
- Blood in the CSF also raises the CSF protein. If the cell count and protein are measured on the same tube of CSF and the peripheral CBC and serum protein are normal, the following guideline is helpful: Subtract 1 mg/dl of protein for every 1,000 RBCs/mm$^3$.

## Cerebrospinal Fluid Findings in Disease States

Table 10-2 lists the CSF findings in normal and disease states. This is general information, and exceptions occur. Most important, normal or minimally abnormal CSF obtained from the lumbar space does not exclude the presence of leptomeningeal tumor. Table 10-3 lists some tumor markers that can be found in the CSF. Diagnosis involves correlating CSF findings with the clinical problem, type and extent of underlying tumor, and results of radiographic studies.

## Pearls and Caveats in Cerebrospinal Fluid Analysis

- CSF should be processed immediately after the sample is obtained to preserve morphology. Cells in the CSF begin to lyse within the first hour and 40% are lysed by 2 hours. This process is minimized by refrigeration.
- Blood in the CSF can be due either to a traumatic lumbar puncture or subarachnoid hemorrhage (SAH). In general, traumatic blood will clear

**Table 10-3**   CSF Tumor Markers

| Tumor Marker | Tumor |
| --- | --- |
| Alpha fetoprotein (AFP) | Teratocarcinoma, yolk sac tumor, embryonal carcinoma |
| Human chorionic gonadotropin, beta subunit (B-HCG) | Choriocarcinoma, embryonal carcinoma |
| Human placental alkaline phosphatase (pALP) | Germinoma |
| Carcinoembryonic antigen (CEA) | Colon cancer |
| CA-125 | Ovarian carcinoma |
| CA 15-3 | Breast cancer |
| Glial fibrillary acidic protein | Gliomas |
| Neuropeptides | Pituitary adenomas |
| B-2 microglobulin | Lymphoma, other malignancies, infection |
| LDH isoenzymes, B glucuronidase | Carcinomas |
| Prostate-specific antigen | Prostate cancer |

during the CSF collection and SAH will not. In SAH, the RBC count in the first tube will be similar to sequential tubes, whereas the count will decrease if the LP was traumatic. An unenhanced CT scan should be done immediately and neurosurgical consultation obtained if there is concern about SAH.

- Obese patients can have an opening pressure of up to 250 mm $H_2O$ in the absence of pathology.

## Suggested Reading

Fishman RA. *Cerebrospinal Fluid in Diseases of the Nervous System* (2nd ed). Philadelphia: W.B. Saunders, 1992.

Patton J. *Neurological Differential Diagnosis.* London: Harold Starke Ltd., 1977.

# 11

# Pathologic Diagnosis

## General Approach

Accurate histologic diagnosis is critical for treatment planning and patient counseling. Surgically obtained tissue usually is required to make a histologic diagnosis. For certain tumors, a definitive diagnosis can be accomplished by vitreous aspirate, cerebrospinal fluid (CSF) cytology, or suggested by the presence of certain tumor markers in the CSF. Tissue is procured by stereotactic (closed) biopsy or by an open procedure, which then may include partial or gross total tumor resection. Ideally, both the neurosurgeon and neuropathologist involved should be experienced in the diagnosis of brain tumors. The neuropathologist should be informed of the location of the tumor and radiographic characteristics. A frozen section is examined intraoperatively, and communication with the pathologist increases the diagnostic value of the tissue obtained. Even when such an approach is used, there is a risk of obtaining nondiagnostic tissue. Sampling error, leading to an erroneously lower grade of tumor or even an incorrect diagnosis, also is possible. Despite the importance of the frozen section, definitive diagnosis always awaits the interpretation of permanent sections.

## Histologic Examination

The specifics of diagnosis of central nervous system (CNS) tumors based on neuropathology can be found in reference texts listed in the Suggested Reading section. Hematoxylin-eosin (H & E) stains are performed on tissue and may be supplemented by a variety of other histologic stains and immunohistochemical investigations, depending on the nature of the suspected tumor. Positive staining for glial fibrillary acidic protein (GFAP) identifies tumors of glial origin. Procedures for estimating the rate of cell proliferation have gained attention recently. One such technique is immunohistochemistry for MIB-1, a monoclonal antibody to a subclone of Ki-67, which is expressed as a labeling index. Of all commercially available proliferation indexes, MIB-1 is favored due to its ability to stain formalin-fixed, paraffin-embedded sections, as well as for its reproducibility. In general, tumors with high MIB-1 labeling indexes tend to behave more aggressively. Long-term data collection in large clinical trials will be necessary to define the significance of this relationship.

Occasionally, electron microscopy is useful for diagnosis, such as the demonstration of cilia in ependymoma cells. Recently, genetic testing has gained importance as a predictor of treatment sensitivity in oligodendrogliomas. Tumors characterized by loss of 1p and 19q are more sensitive to treatment, compared to those that lack these genetic features.

## Suggested Reading

Bigner DD, McLendon RE, and Bruner JM (eds). *Russell and Rubinstein's Pathology of Tumors of the Nervous System* (6th ed). New York: Oxford University Press, 1998.

Burger PC, Scheithauer BW. *Atlas of Tumor Pathology: Tumors of the Central Nervous System.* Third Series. Fascicle 10. Bethesda, MD: Armed Forces Institute of Pathology, 1993.

Kleihues P, Cavanee WK (eds). *Pathology and Genetics of Tumors of the Nervous System* (2nd ed). New York: Oxford University Press, 2000.

Schold SC Jr, Burger PC, Mendelsohn DB, et al. *Primary Tumors of the Brain and Spinal Cord.* Boston: Butterworth–Heinemann, 1997.

# IV

## Commonly Used Treatments in Neuro-Oncology

# 12

# Radiotherapy

Radiotherapy is an important treatment for central nervous system (CNS) tumors and has been demonstrated to extend survival and improve the quality of life for patients with many of the primary and metastatic brain tumors. Although most patients tolerate the acute phase of brain irradiation reasonably well, significant subacute and chronic side effects can be associated with therapy. Neurologic structures also are subject to injury due to radiotherapy applied as treatment for non–central nervous system tumors. For example, neck irradiation can accelerate atherosclerosis of the internal carotid artery. Basic information regarding radiotherapy and its effects on the CNS and peripheral nervous system are summarized in this chapter.

## Basic Terms

- *Gy* is the absorbed dose of radiation: 1 Gy = 1 joule/kg = 100 rad.
- *Fraction* is the dose in Gy of radiation administered at each treatment setting.
- *Field* specifies the specific volume of irradiated tissue.
- *Teletherapy* is an external-beam radiotherapy from a source located at a distance from the patient (orthovoltage or supervoltage machines).
- In *brachytherapy*, the radiation source is placed within or in close proximity to the tumor tissue, usually in the form of radioactive seeds.
- *Radiotherapy planning* includes considering treatment options, localizing precisely the tumor tissue, identifying the target volume, planning for proper immobilization, constructing blocks to shield certain tissues, and marking superficial skin ("tattoos") to ensure consistent positioning. Plans for the proper immobilization of children and uncooperative patients may include sedation or anesthesia.

- The radiotherapy plan is *simulated* using superficial radiation that can produce direct images and radiographs to confirm the accuracy of the treatment plan.

## Treatment Strategies in Neuro-Oncology

### External-Beam Radiotherapy

External-beam radiotherapy most commonly is delivered via photon beams from a linear accelerator. Radiation oncologists and physicists design treatment plans based on the size, location, geometry, and anticipated biologic behavior of the tumor. The basic strategy is to maximize the dose to involved tissue and minimize the dose to surrounding tissues. For tumors that are diffusely infiltrative, such as primary CNS lymphoma and most gliomas, there are significant issues regarding the definition of tumor margins and the problem of the radiographically normal or nonenhancing tumor. Therefore, for most CNS tumors, treatment encompasses "bulky" disease (as defined by contrast-enhanced computed tomography [CT] or magnetic resonance imaging [MRI] scans) and microscopic disease presumed to be present.

### Brachytherapy

Most of the experience using brachytherapy for intracranial tumors has been with the use of $I^{131}$ impregnated seeds. Restrictions include the size, geometry, and location of the tumor and the need for craniotomy. Brachytherapy largely has been abandoned because of a lack of evidence that it yields a superior outcome compared with external-beam radiotherapy. Furthermore, radiation necrosis occurs in about half of patients following brachytherapy, often necessitating surgical removal of the affected tissue.

### Hyperfractionation

Reducing the fraction size and increasing the number of fractions has been explored in clinical trials as an effort to improve tumor control and decrease neurologic morbidity. To date, hyperfractionation has not proven superior to standard single daily fractions.

### Radiosurgery

Radiosurgery is performed with a focused, high dose-per-fraction beam directed to small intracranial masses, using either multiple cobalt beams (gamma knife) or a linear accelerator. Newer methods using multileaf collimators (e.g., Novalis® system) allow for precise shaped-beam treatments.

### Radiosensitizers

Radiosensitizers are agents that sensitize tumor cells to the effects of radiotherapy.

## Adverse Effects of Radiotherapy

- Adverse effects of radiotherapy can occur either during or following treatment.
- Acute side effects tend to be reversible, respond to corticosteroids, and do not necessarily correlate with the subsequent occurrence of long-term side effects.
- Available radiation tolerance data includes a range of tolerances of CNS tissue. Therefore, toxicity may be seen at or below "tolerance doses" in individual patients.
- In general, the risk of toxicity increases with larger fraction size, higher total dose, and larger treatment volumes. Comorbidities, such as diabetes mellitus, hypertension, and advanced age, probably also increase the risk.
- It is as difficult to predict the occurrence of toxicity as it is to predict treatment response for individual patients.
- Determining the causative role of radiotherapy in the occurrence of late toxicity is difficult. Patients who survive long enough to develop toxicity usually have received other therapies such as chemotherapy and one or more surgeries. Terms such as *radiation necrosis* and *radiation injury* typically have been used to describe such complications, but the term *treatment effect* is perhaps more accurate and appropriate and recognizes the possible contributions of other therapies.
- Specific tumor types may play a role in determining the risk for neurologic injury. For example, patients with primary CNS lymphoma are exquisitely sensitive to the adverse effects of combined modality therapies, perhaps because of the perivascular nature of the disease.
- Specific side effects based on the structures treated are summarized next.

## Brain

### Acute Effects

- Although most patients tolerate the acute phase of brain irradiation with modest difficulty, the effects vary among individuals. Some patients can continue most of their normal activities, whereas other patients may be significantly impaired during treatment.

- Most patients experience some degree of fatigue and alopecia.
- Other common symptoms include headache, nausea or vomiting, anorexia, and worsening of neurologic deficits related to the location of the tumor.
- Most radiation oncologists recommend the use of corticosteroids during radiotherapy and the dose is tapered after completion of treatment.
- When neurologic symptoms develop they usually are manageable by raising the corticosteroid dose.
- Patients with larger tumors that are associated with significant mass effect can develop an increase in intracranial pressure (ICP) resulting in worsening neurologic deficit, increased somnolence, and other signs and symptoms of increased ICP. Occasionally, such patients require hospitalization for management of raised ICP and associated neurologic deficits. This should not be construed as tumor progression or radiation failure.

### Early-Delayed Radiation Encephalopathy

This syndrome occurs 1–4 months following radiotherapy, characterized by a deterioration in neurologic status that may include focal or generalized signs and symptoms. Differential diagnosis between early-delayed radiation encephalopathy and tumor progression is difficult to make on clinical grounds. CT and MRI scans may demonstrate an increase in enhancement or an increase in mass effect, further confusing the picture. Positron emission tomography (PET) scans reveal an area of hypometabolism in cases of radiation effect. Signs and symptoms improve by 6 months and symptomatic improvement is associated with corticosteroid therapy. Short-term memory may be impaired in the weeks immediately following radiotherapy and generally improves 4–8 months later.

### Delayed Radiation Effects: Leukoencephalopathy and Necrosis

*Leukoencephalopathy* refers to the late effects of cranial irradiation, which typically result in white matter injury causing deficits of cognitive function. The extent of involvement ranges from mild to severe. Mildly affected patients may have deficits in short-term memory and cognitive processing that still permit independent function. Severely affected patients develop marked cognitive deficits, frank dementia, and ataxia. Areas of increased signal intensity are seen in the white matter on T2 MRI, but the extent of these radiographic findings does not correlate directly with the severity of clinical impairment. Severely affected patients are found to have marked white matter changes on MRI, atrophy, and communicating hydrocephalus. A subset of these patients may benefit from ventriculoperitoneal shunting.

*Radiation necrosis* has been reported as early as 3–4 months and as late as 20 years following therapeutic cranial irradiation. The patient may develop neurologic signs and symptoms that are referable to the irradiated area of brain. Radiation necrosis is visualized on CT or MRI scans as a new area of enhancement, which commonly is ring-like. As with early-delayed radiation encephalopathy, distinguishing radiation necrosis from tumor recurrence by CT or MRI scanning is unreliable, but positron emission tomography (PET) scanning often is helpful. Reviewing the radiographic studies with the radiation oncologist is critical in determining whether the new abnormality is within the previously irradiated area. Definitive diagnosis requires biopsy. However, specimens may be difficult to interpret as both radiation necrosis and tumor may be found. Steroids may provide palliation of symptoms but steroid response does not distinguish between radiation necrosis and tumor recurrence.

## Spinal Cord

### Acute Radiation Myelopathy

Worsening of neurologic deficit during radiotherapy usually is mild to moderate in severity. The process is self-limiting, and symptoms generally are improved by temporarily increasing the corticosteroid dose. This phenomenon occurs primarily in patients with intrinsic spinal cord tumors but may occur with epidural metastases.

### Early-Delayed Radiation Myelopathy

Early-delayed radiation myelopathy is a phenomenon due to transient demyelination of the irradiated spinal cord, producing Lhermitte's sign. The peak time of onset is 4 months following radiation and symptoms generally are limited to Lhermitte's sign. Associated neurologic deficit is uncommon. Other causes of Lhermitte's sign should be considered (see Chapter 5), and the affected portion of the spinal cord should be imaged with MRI if there is associated neurologic deficit or a change in the neurologic examination. This process is self-limiting, and symptoms generally abate within 6 months. Steroids are helpful in attenuating the Lhermitte's sign in patients who find it distressing.

### Delayed Radiation Myelopathy

Delayed radiation myelopathy occurs with a peak onset at 14 months following radiotherapy. The onset of symptoms ranges from subacute to rapid. Dysesthesias are the most common presenting symptoms and paresis below the level of the lesion may follow, along with difficulties with urinary or anal sphincter function. Symptoms typically worsen initially, then stabilize; and this process usually is irreversible. The differential diagnosis includes tumor recurrence, second tumor formation (radiation-induced tumor), and unrelated processes. The spine should be imaged to help define the etiology of the patient's symptoms.

## Craniospinal Irradiation

Combined cranial and spinal irradiation typically is used for patients with tumors that tend to disseminate within the neuraxis and provides curative therapy for some of these tumors. Typically an intermediate dose (e.g., 36 Gy) is administered to the entire neuraxis and a higher dose (e.g., 55 Gy) is given as a boost to the primary site. Craniospinal irradiation carries with it all the potential risks of both cranial and spinal radiotherapy discussed previously, and the course of craniospinal irradiation may be more difficult for patients to tolerate. Due to the large volume of tissue treated, symptoms of fatigue, nausea or vomiting, and anorexia occur with increased frequency. Myelosuppression is common because of the large volume of bone marrow irradiated. However, because the risk of radiation injury is dose related, areas of the neuraxis that receive the lower dose are less at risk for late effects such as myelopathy.

## Brachial and Lumbar Plexus

The brachial and lumbar plexuses are at risk for injury following radiotherapy when they are encompassed in a treatment field for nonneurologic tumors. Typical examples include regional radiotherapy for breast cancer and pelvic/abdominal radiotherapy for lymphoma, gastrointestinal, or gynecologic tumors. Refer to Chapter 48 for a discussion of plexopathies including those due to radiotherapy.

## Cranial Nerves

The cranial nerves are relatively resistant to radiation-induced injury. Cranial nerves (CN) I (olfactory nerve) and VIII (auditory nerve) are the most commonly affected during radiotherapy. When the ear and pathways of CN VIII are included in the radiotherapy port, tinnitus and hearing loss during or immediately following radiotherapy are common. While this can be due to direct toxicity to CN VIII, more commonly it relates to serous otitis. Refer to Chapters 34 and 52 for further information.

## Pituitary Gland and Hypothalamus

Endocrine aberrations are fairly common following radiotherapy to the pituitary region or hypothalamus. Patients with pituitary tumors or pituitary surgery are particularly vulnerable. Endocrine abnormalities also occur following prophylactic whole-brain radiotherapy, such as is used for small-cell lung cancer. Aberrations of one or more hormone pathways can occur. Comprehensive endocrine evaluation is indicated in patients with suspected radiation-induced pituitary or hypothalamic injury to determine the specific hormones affected and the strategy for replacement.

- *Growth hormone* is the pituitary hormone most sensitive to radiotherapy. Children commonly manifest decreased growth following cranial irradiation.
- *LH* (luteinizing hormone) and *FSH* (follicle-stimulating hormone) deficiencies following radiotherapy can result in irregular menses, amenorrhea, sexual difficulties, and decreased libido. Measurement of serum FSH, LH, progesterone, and estrogen levels in women helps guide replacement therapy. In men, when serum testosterone levels are low, replacement may improve symptoms.
- *TSH* (thyroid-stimulating hormone) deficiency results in central hypothyroidism. Serum TSH and T4 levels are low, as compared with primary hypothyroidism in which serum TSH is elevated.
- *ACTH* (adrenocorticotropic hormone) deficiency results in central adrenal failure. Although this is uncommon, the hypothalamic/ adrenal axis should be evaluated prior to treatment of specific pituitary hormone deficiencies. Specifically, replacement of thyroid hormone in the setting of undiagnosed adrenal failure can precipitate a life-threatening adrenal crisis.
- *Panhypopituitarism* may follow pituitary region radiotherapy and present months to years later.

## Peripheral Nerves

The peripheral nerves are relatively radioresistant. Alternative explanations should be sought for peripheral nerve symptoms in cancer patients (see Chapter 48).

## Radiation-Induced Tumors

Radiation-induced tumors can follow therapeutic radiotherapy to the nervous system for primary CNS tumors, metastatic tumors, prophylaxis for brain metastasis, or unavoidable CNS radiation as a result of treatment of tumors located near the nervous system. A radiation-induced tumor of the CNS should be considered when the tumor is of a different histology than the original tumor and the new tumor is located within previously radiated CNS tissue. A delay of 4–20 years is most typical. The best-established examples include meningiomas, sarcomas, and malignant peripheral nerve sheath tumors.

### Suggested Reading

Gregor A, Cull A, Traynor E, et al. Neuropsychometric evaluation of long-term survivors of adult brain tumours: relationship with tumour and treatment parameters. *Radiother Oncol.* 1996;41(1):55–59.

Leibel SA, Phillips TL. *Textbook of Radiation Oncology.* Philadelphia: W.B. Saunders, 1998.

Leibel SA, Sheline GE. Radiation therapy for neoplasms of the brain. *J Neurosurg.* 1987;66(1):1–22.

Thiessen B, DeAngelis LM. Hydrocephalus in radiation leukoencephalopathy: Results of ventriculoperitoneal shunting. *Arch Neurol.* 1998;55(5):705–710.

# 13

# Chemotherapy

Chemotherapy, or the use of drugs in the treatment of cancer, can lead to the long-term control of many malignancies. Some tumors, such as testicular cancer or Hodgkin's disease, may be cured even when they are widespread. Others, such as pancreatic or gastric cancer, are only minimally responsive to drug treatment. Central nervous system (CNS) neoplasms may be controlled by chemotherapy, although cure is not the usual expectation. Typically, chemotherapy for CNS malignancy serves as an adjunct to surgical or radiation therapy. It also may be used for tumors that progress after primary treatment.

As chemotherapy may be associated with severe toxicity, it should be given under the supervision of one skilled in the administration and monitoring of such agents. Some of these agents are discussed in Table 13-1. Typically, therapy is initiated at a specialized center but requires detailed and close communication with physicians in referring facilities, as it is not always practical to travel to the treating center for every problem.

**Table 13-1**  Some Useful Chemotherapeutic Agents in the Treatment of CNS Neoplasms

| Agent | Uses | Route | Dose Range | Major Side Effects | Considerations |
|---|---|---|---|---|---|
| Carmustine (BCNU) | Malignant glioma | IV | 240 mg/m² over 3 d q 6–8 wks | Nausea<br>Myelosuppression<br>Pulmonary fibrosis (greatest at cumulative doses >1400 mg/m²) | Platelet nadir may be prolonged<br>Myelosuppression is cumulative<br>Leukemogenic |
| Lomustine (CCNU) | Malignant glioma, oligodendroglioma | PO | 110 mg/m² q 6 wk | Nausea<br>Myelosuppression<br>Pulmonary fibrosis (greatest at cumulative doses >1100 mg/m²) | Platelet nadir may be prolonged<br>Myelosuppression is cumulative<br>Leukemogenic |
| Procarbazine | Malignant glioma, oligodendroglioma | PO | Varies | CNS depression<br>Peripheral neuropathy<br>Myelosuppression | Many drug interactions, including disulfuram-like effect with ethanol<br>Avoid tyramine-rich foods<br>Leukemogenic |
| Temozolomide | Malignant glioma | PO | 150–200 mg/m²/d × 5 d q 4 wks | Nausea<br>Headache<br>Fatigue<br>Myelosuppression<br>Constipation | |

| | | | | | |
|---|---|---|---|---|---|
| Vincristine | Malignant glioma, oligodendroglioma | IV | 1 mg/m² (max = 2 mg) q wk | Peripheral neuropathy<br>Constipation<br>Vesicant | Beware of extravasation |
| Cisplatin | Malignant glioma, PNET | IV | 25–100 mg/m² q 1–3 wks | Nausea<br>Renal insufficiency<br>Peripheral neuropathy<br>Myelosuppression | Strongly emetogenic<br>Aggressive use of fluids minimizes nephrotoxicity |
| Cyclophosphamide | Medulloblastoma | IV, PO | Varies with regimen | Nausea<br>Myelosuppression | Leukemogenic |
| Irinotecan | Malignant glioma | IV | 125 mg/m²/wk × 6 wks | Severe diarrhea<br>Nausea<br>Myelosuppression | |

IV, intravenous; PO, oral; PNET, primitive neuroectodermal tumor.

## Patient Education

Before treatment is given, detailed patient and family education is indicated, including

- Indications for therapy.
- Scheduling of therapy.
- Potential side effects.
- Potential benefits.
- How drug antitumor effect will be monitored.
- Logisitics of therapy:
  - Where it will be given.
  - By what route will it be administered.
  - When required blood tests will be drawn.
  - Who will be available should problems or questions arise.

## Goals of Therapy

The expectations for treatment must be clear. Is it to be given as an adjunct to enhance the efficacy of radiation? Is it being used with palliative intent? Will it be used with the expectation of increasing survival? When the endpoint is defined, it should be discussed with the patient and their family. For example, if a tumor is being treated with palliative intent, the symptoms to be palliated should be specified. The method to assess objective tumor response should be clarified. *The original goals should be revisited often to determine if they have been achieved with acceptable toxicity.*

## Complications of Chemotherapy

Most chemotherapy regimens are associated with some potential toxicity. These can be grouped into those that cause symptomatic discomfort and those that are potentially dangerous. Management of these problems is discussed in other chapters.

Uncomfortable symptoms include

- Nausea and vomiting.
- Alopecia.
- Mucositis.
- Alterations in bowel function.
- Fatigue.

Potentially life-threatening symptoms include

- Neutropenia.
- Thrombocytopenia.

- Pulmonary complications.
- CNS complications.
- Hypersensitivity reactions.

Although chemotherapy for CNS neoplasms often consists of single-agent therapy given with radiotherapy, combination chemotherapy is used increasingly. A commonly used regimen, termed *PCV*, consists of

Lomustine: 110 mg/m$^2$ PO, d 1 (or divided d 1–2)
Procarbazine: 60 mg/m$^2$ PO, d 8–21
Vincristine: 1.4 mg/m$^2$ IV, d 8 and 29 (maximum of 2 mg/dose)

## Investigative Therapy

Chemotherapy, as it is currently used in the management of CNS malignancy, remains limited. For any patient in whom treatment is contemplated, entry into a well-designed clinical trial always is a reasonable option. Such trials offer patients the potential for improved therapy under carefully monitored conditions.

## Suggested Reading

Bower M, Newlands ES, Bleehen NM, et al. Multicenter CRC phase II trial of temozolomide in recurrent or progressive high-grade glioma. *Cancer Chemother Pharmacol.* 1997;40:484.

EORTC Brain Tumor Group. Effect of CCNU on survival of objective remission and duration of free interval in patients with malignant brain glioma: Final evaluation. *Eur J Cancer.* 1978;14:851.

Fine HA, Dear KBG, Loeffler JS, et al. Meta-analysis of radiation therapy with and without adjuvant chemotherapy for malignant gliomas in adults. *Cancer.* 1993;71:2585.

Green SB, Byar DP, Walker MD, et al. Comparison of carmustine, procarbazine, and high-dose methylprednisolone as additions to surgery and radiotherapy for the treatment of malignant glioma. *Cancer Treat Rep.* 1983;67:1.

Levin VA, Silver P, Hannigan J, et al. Superiority of post-radiotherapy adjuvant chemotherapy with CCNU, procarbazine, and vincristine (PCV) over BCNU for anaplastic gliomas: NCOG 6G61: Final report. *Int J Radiat Oncol Biol Phys.* 1990;18:321.

Rodriquez LA, Prados M, Silver P, Levin VA. Re-evaluation of procarbazine for the treatment of recurrent malignant CNS tumors. *Cancer.* 1989;64.

Rosenbloom ML, Reynolds AF, Smith KA, et al. Chloroethyl-cyclohexyl-nitrosourea (CCNU) in the treatment of malignant brain tumors. *Int J Radiat Oncol Biol Phys.* 1973;39:306.

Walker MD, Green SB, Byar DP, et al. Randomized comparison of radiotherapy and nitrosoureas for the treatment of malignant glioma after surgery. *N Engl J Med.* 1980;303:1323.

# 14

# Corticosteroids

Corticosteroids (CS) are commonly used in patients with a variety of neuro-oncologic conditions. Following the initial diagnosis of a primary or metastatic brain tumor, CS treatment often is required to control symptoms related to increased intracranial pressure (ICP) or peritumoral edema. Continued CS treatment is needed in selected patients to alleviate neurologic deficits or symptoms related to increased ICP. Many patients develop acute or chronic undesirable side effects during CS therapy.

## Mechanism of Action

- CS counteract vasogenic edema by decreasing the permeability of central nervous system (CNS) endothelial tight junctions (the blood-brain barrier).
- CS exert a direct cytotoxic effect in lymphomas, including those within the brain.

## Presteroid Evaluation

The following evaluations are suggested prior to initiating CS therapy or shortly thereafter:

- Complete medical history and physical examination with particular attention to
  - Previous corticosteroid treatment: indication, side effects, tolerance.
  - Signs or symptoms of acute or chronic infection, tuberculosis (TB) status or exposure.
  - History of psychosis or other psychological problems.
  - Individual and family history of diabetes, including gestational diabetes.
  - Evidence of pre-existing osteoporosis.
  - History of peptic ulcer disease.
  - Presence of obesity.

– History of hypertension or cardiovascular disease.
– Medication review.
- Laboratory investigations: electrolytes, blood urea nitrogen (BUN)/ creatinine, calcium, magnesium, glucose, hepatic profile, complete blood count.
- Anticonvulsant levels (the addition of CS can alter anticonvulsant levels).
- Chest X ray or purified protein derivative (PPD) test.

## Dosing Indications and Guidelines

Dexamethasone (DEX) is the corticosteroid most commonly used in neuro-oncology. DEX has a long half-life and theoretically can be dosed once daily. In practice, the dose typically is divided bid to qid for improved gastrointestinal tolerance. The timing of doses should be scheduled during waking hours to avoid unnecessary interruption of sleep.

- Many patients require CS at the time of diagnosis of a primary or metastatic brain tumor. Consider CS therapy when there are
  – Significant peritumoral edema or mass effect radiographically.
  – Radiographic or clinical signs of cerebral herniation.
  – Significant neurologic deficits or symptoms related to peritumoral edema or increased ICP.
- A typical starting dose of DEX for patients with significant peritumoral edema is 6 mg qid. In some patients, a "loading dose" of 10–20 mg also is given.
- Selected patients may require higher initial doses, particularly within the first 24–48 hours of treatment. Although it is best to minimize the total dose and duration of CS therapy, it is preferable to overtreat initially than undertreat. This is especially critical during the initial management and evaluation of patients with suspected spinal cord compression.
- Perioperatively, CS generally are administered before biopsy or resection. When significant mass effect is present, CS should be started 24–48 hours before surgery, if possible.
- CS are part of the acute management of herniation syndromes as outlined in Chapter 43.
- CS are part of the acute management of spinal cord compression as outlined in Chapter 27.
- CS can be helpful as adjunctive pain therapy to opiates for cancer pain, particularly when tumor involvement is near or within neural structures.

## Side Effects and Management

Potential side effects of CS therapy must be weighed against potential benefits on an individual patient basis. The degree and number of

CS-related side effects varies greatly from patient to patient. Whereas certain side effects may severely limit CS use (e.g., uncontrollable hyperglycemia or psychosis), most others are more manageable. Because the side effects of CS therapy can impair the patient's quality of life and present life-threatening risks, it is important to minimize the total duration and dose as much as possible. Patients and their caregivers should be educated regarding the potential side effects of CS treatment. Common side effects such as constipation, insomnia, and appetite stimulation are best managed in a pre-emptive fashion. Table 14-1 depicts the more common side effects and strategies for their management.

**Table 14-1**   Corticosteroid Side Effects and Management

| Organ System and Clinical Problem | Strategies for Management and Follow-up Care |
|---|---|
| **Immune function** | Increased risk of infections |
| **Pulmonary** | Risk of infections including PCP |
| **Cardiac** | Exacerbation of CHF, edema, hypertension, angina |
| **Dermatologic** | |
| Acneiform rash<br>  Patient discomfort and embarrassment<br>  Risk of secondary skin infections | Keep skin clean and dry, apply topical erythromycin ointment, wash affected areas with low strength benzoyl peroxide |
| Attenuation of rashes due to other drugs | High index of clinical suspicion for drug rashes, especially during taper of steroids |
| Flushing, night sweats | Replacement estrogen as appropriate Loose cotton clothing and bedding |
| Skin thinning and breakdown (chronic use) | Strategies to protect skin and prevent pressure sores |
| Hair thinning | |
| **Renal and urinary** | |
| Polyurea, polydipsia | Check for hyperglycemia, hypo- or hypernatremia, urinary tract infection |
| Nocturia | Midday low dose diuretic, elevate legs for 1–2 hours before going to bed, exclude UTI or prostatic enlargement |
| **Metabolic and endocrine** | |
| Impaired glucose tolerance, diabetic state | Dietary counseling, ADA diet, avoidance of simple sugars, oral hypoglycemic agents, insulin |

*continues*

**Table 14-1**   Corticosteroid Side Effects and Management   *continued*

| Organ System and Clinical Problem | Strategies for Management and Follow-up Care |
| --- | --- |
| Thyroid | May inhibit TSH secretion |
| Appetite stimulation, weight gain | Dietary counseling, monitor weight |
| Potassium wasting | Supplemental potassium |
| **Gastrointestinal** | |
| Nausea, GI upset, heartburn | Antacids, H-2 blockers |
| Peptic ulcer disease | Prophylaxis for selected patients |
| Constipation | Stool softeners, laxatives, increase bulk fiber in diet and fluid intake |
| **Neurobehavioral** | |
| Agitation, hyperactivity, irritability, mania, psychosis | Pharmacologic therapy: respiridone |
| Insomnia | Time CS doses early in the day Pharmacologic therapy: ambien |
| Depression | Antidepressant therapy: tricyclic anti-depressant agents, SSRI |
| **Neurologic and neuromuscular** | |
| Proximal muscle weakness (myopathy) | Increase mobility, physical therapy |
| Headache | Consider pseudotumor cerebri |
| **Bone** | |
| Osteoporosis | Calcium, vitamin D supplementation Encourage weight bearing exercise Estrogen replacement (postmenopausal) |
| Vertebral body compression fractures | Evaluated back pain, exclude metastatic disease |
| Aseptic necrosis (femoral or humeral head) | |
| **Pharmacologic multiple drug interactions** | CS can decrease: some anticonvulsant levels, effects of coumadin CS can increase: cyclosporin Increases CS metabolism: phenytoin, rifampin, phenobarbital, ephedrine |
| Steroid withdrawal syndrome (myalgia, arthralgia, lethargy, low grade fever, nausea, vomiting, anorexia, postural hypotension, headache, papilledema/ pseudotumor cerebri, adrenal insuffi-ciency, adrenal crisis) | Taper off more slowly, evaluate for adrenal insufficiency |

PCP, *Pneumocystis carinii* pneumonia; CHF, congestive heart failure; UTI, urinary tract infection; ADA, American Diabetes Association; TSH, thyroid stimulating hormone; GI, gastrointestinal; SSRI, selective seratonin reuptake inhibitor.

## Pearls and Pitfalls

- CS can reduce the amount of contrast enhancement on computed tomography (CT) and magnetic resonance imaging (MRI) studies.
- The peak therapeutic effect of CS therapy may not occur for 24–72 hours.
- Patients already on maintenance CS therapy tend not to respond to small increases in doses. A helpful guideline is to double the daily dose and then taper the dose based on the clinical response.
- Withdrawing ("tapering") CS therapy must be individualized based on the patient's neurologic symptoms, degree of residual mass effect radiographically, and ongoing side effects. Furthermore, once the taper is designed and implemented, ongoing re-evaluation is needed.
- CS therapy does not improve symptoms related to irreversible brain destruction (from tumor or secondary brain infarction) or surgical deficits.
- Adrenal insufficiency can develop following CS administration and withdrawal. Even patients remaining on low doses of CS can develop adrenal insufficiency when stressed. Therefore, such patients require "stress doses" of CS at times of systemic illness, vomiting, and the perioperative period.

# 15

# Neurosurgical
# Interventions

Neurosurgical intervention is warranted in almost all cases of primary central nervous system (CNS) tumors and for many metastatic tumors. A biopsy usually establishes a definitive histologic diagnosis and resection generally provides palliation of symptoms or definitive therapy. The role of surgery depends on the nature of the tumor, and further details can be found in the chapters on specific tumors. With modern neurosurgical techniques, most patients with extra-axial brain tumors are cured with minimal residual neurologic deficit. A few parenchymal brain tumors can be cured surgically, and extensive resection of parenchymal brain tumors is becoming increasingly safe and well tolerated. Debulking parenchymal brain tumors often improves the patient's quality of life by reducing symptoms related to increased intracranial pressure (ICP) or focal deficits, and the requirement for corticosteroids may be reduced as well. However, due to their infiltrating nature, complete surgical resection of parenchymal brain tumors generally is not possible. Furthermore, some tumors are not resectable because of diffuse brain infiltration or encasement of vital structures. Examples include intrinsic pontine gliomas, optic chiasm and hypothalamic gliomas, tumors invading the cavernous sinus, and tumors encasing large intracranial arteries. The more commonly used neurosurgical procedures are outlined in this chapter.

## Stereotactic Biopsy

Stereotactic biopsy (SB) is commonly performed to obtain tissue for pathologic analysis and can be performed through a small opening in the skull (burr hole) or as an open procedure. SB involves localizing the target lesion with the use of computed tomography (CT) or magnetic resonance imaging (MRI) guidance. The target is the area of enhancing tumor on CT or MRI scan or the abnormal MRI T2 signal area in cases of nonenhancing tumors. An external frame, which is fixed to the patient's head, is used to provide radiographic guidance. Recently, frameless systems using fiduciary markers attached to the patient's head have been developed and are being used to guide sterotactic biopsies and resections.

## Stereotactic-Guided Volumetric Resections

Stereotactic-guided volumetric resections use CT or MRI guidance and intraoperative video for precise localization and resection of tumor tissue.

## Functional Mapping and Electrocorticography

Functional mapping is performed on selected patients at the time of craniotomy. Direct electrical stimulation of cortical structures identifies areas of functional cortex and resection of these areas is avoided. Electrocorticography is the technique of intraoperative recording of seizure foci to identify epileptogenic areas of brain.

## Ventriculoperitoneal Shunts and External Ventricular Drains

Ventriculoperitoneal (VP) shunts and external ventricular drains (EVD) are methods of diverting cerebrospinal fluid (CSF) from the ventricles to manage hydrocephalus. EVD also are used acutely to manage some patients with increased ICP. Most often, the frontal horn of the right lateral ventricle is chosen for placement of the drain or shunt. An EVD is used as a temporary intervention and diverts CSF to an external collection device. A VP shunt is a more definitive procedure and involves placement of a subcutaneous catheter into the peritoneal space.

# V

## Specific Tumors

# 16

# Malignant Astrocytomas

Malignant astrocytomas are the most common primary brain tumors in adults. Both subtypes, anaplastic astrocytomas (AA) and glioblastoma multiforme (GBM), are diffusely infiltrative central nervous system (CNS) tumors. There is good evidence that the tumor grade (AA vs. GBM) affects patient survival. Commonly used treatments include surgery, radiotherapy, and chemotherapy. Almost all patients will relapse following initial therapy, and investigational modalities are important therapeutic options for such patients. Supportive therapies, management of neurologic deficits, and treatment of related symptoms, such as seizures, are important in optimizing the patient's quality of life.

## Synonyms and Classification

- Although the term *glioma* technically encompasses any tumor of glial cell origin, it frequently is used incorrectly as a synonym for astrocytoma.
- Glioblastoma (glioblastoma multiforme) is a World Health Organization (WHO) grade IV astrocytoma.
- Anaplastic astrocytoma is a WHO grade III astrocytoma.
- Gliosarcoma is a tumor composed of both astrocytic and sarcomatous elements and has a prognosis similar to GBM.

## Cell of Origin

Both arise from CNS astrocytes.

## Incidence

- Glioblastoma: 2.6/100,000 person-years; 22.6% of primary intracranial tumors.
- Anaplastic astrocytoma: 0.48/100,000 person-years; 4.3% of primary intracranial tumors.

## Mean Age at Diagnosis

- Glioblastoma: 62 years.
- Anaplastic astrocytoma: 50 years.

## Typical Locations

Malignant astrocytomas typically are found in the cerebral hemispheres, brain stem, or thalamus. Cerebellar hemisphere involvement is uncommon in adults but common in children.

## Presentation

Signs and symptoms of an intracranial lesion are discussed in Chapter 4. Seizures and headaches are common presenting symptoms. Loss of initiative and personality and cognitive changes also are common.

## Radiographic Appearance

- Computed tomography (CT)
  - Hypodense on nonenhanced images with hyperdense areas if hemorrhage has occurred.
  - Contrast enhancement usually is ring-like or heterogeneous.
  - Central necrosis, manifested by an area of marked hypodensity, often is present.
  - Calcification is uncommon and suggests a lower-grade astrocytoma or oligodendroglioma.
- Magnetic resonance imaging (MRI)
  - Hypointense on unenhanced T1 images.
  - Contrast enhancement usually is ring-like or heterogeneous.
  - Mild to extensive surrounding white matter abnormalities characterized by increased signal intensity on T2 images. This characteristic represents both vasogenic edema and infiltrating tumor.

## Pathology

Gross examination reveals grayish pink tumor tissue that is soft and often granular. A peripheral rim may be present but no defined capsule. A central area of softening often is present and may include necrotic tissue or hemorrhagic changes. Microscopic examination reveals some or all of the following features: increased cellularity, nuclear and cytoplasmic pleomorphism, mitotic figures, endothelial proliferation, and necrosis. These features are used for histologic grading and the presence of necrosis in a nonirradiated tumor specimen distinguishes GBM from AA. Table 16-1 lists the grading schemes that have been in widespread use for astrocytomas during the past few decades. Variability of pathologic features within a tumor specimen is common and sampling error can cause inaccurate grading. The grade is based on the most malignant appearing portion of the specimen.

## Nervous System Staging

A detailed neurologic history and examination is obtained. A cranial MRI scan is obtained.

## Systemic Staging

Systemic metastases are rare. Systemic symptoms usually are due to unrelated medical problems or systemic complications of treatment and should be evaluated as clinically indicated.

**Table 16-1**    Pathologic Grading of Fibrillary Astrocytic Tumors

| Kernohan | Ringertz-Burger-Vogel | St. Anne–Mayo | WHO |
| --- | --- | --- | --- |
| I | Astrocytoma | 0 criteria[a] | II[b] |
| II | Anaplastic astrocytoma | 1 criteria | III |
| III | Glioblastoma | 2 criteria | IV |
| IV | Glioblastoma | 3 or 4 criteria | IV |

WHO, World Health Organization.

[a]Histologic criteria for the St. Anne–Mayo system include cellular atypia, endothelial proliferation, and mitotic activity.

[b]WHO grade I is reserved for atypical astrocytomas, such as pilocytic astrocytomas.

## Usual Treatment

- *Surgery* provides a diagnosis, may relieve symptoms, and may prolong survival.
- *Maximal resection* removes the most tumor possible while preserving neurologic function. Retrospective reviews support the concept that such an approach improves survival and time to tumor recurrence. This approach also reduces symptoms of increased intracranial pressure (ICP), reduces corticosteroid dependence, and thus enhances the patient's quality of life. The use of surgery at recurrence must be individualized. Selected patients may benefit.
- *Radiotherapy* has been found effective in large, randomized studies to significantly prolong survival. Doses of about 6000 cGy are given over 6 to 7 weeks. The tumor, as defined on T2 image, and a surrounding margin are treated.
- The role of *stereotactic radiosurgery (SRS) boost* remains undefined and may increase the risk of radiation necrosis.
- *Chemotherapy* at the time of diagnosis increases the number of long-term survivors and may prolong overall survival and delay recurrence. The favorable effects of chemotherapy are most notable in younger patients. When given at recurrence, chemotherapy can provide temporary responses and extend survival for some patients.
- The most widely used treatment approach at diagnosis is radiotherapy with or without nitrosourea (NU) based chemotherapy. The two NU-based regimens commonly used are BCNU (carmustine) and PCV (procarbazine, CCNU [lomustine], vincristine). Although conflicting data exist regarding which regimen is more favorable, BCNU generally is better tolerated than PCV.
- There is minimal evidence to support the use of postirradiation chemotherapy with standard agents in patients over the age of 65.

## Outcome

Median survival is defined as the time point when 50% of patients have died. For GBM, median survival with supportive treatment is limited to 8–12 weeks, and aggressive therapy with radiation and chemotherapy extends this to 48–54 weeks. For AA, a median survival of 3 years can be expected with aggressive therapy. Although the outcome also relates to several prognostic factors, which follow, predicting outcomes for individual patients is difficult.

- Tumor grade: AA vs. GBM.
- Age: The most important prognostic indicator for malignant astrocytoma other than grade is age. Patients under age 40 survive longer than

those over age 40. Patients over age 65 usually have short survival lasting a median of 6 months.

- Performance status: In general, patients with better performance status survive longer. This is usually measured as the Karnofsky Performance Score (KPS, see Appendix 2).
- Sex: Women may have a slight survival advantage.

## Areas of Investigation

- Sequencing chemotherapy before radiotherapy, dose intensification, radiosensitizers, non-nitrosourea-based chemotherapy regimens, intra-arterial chemotherapy, angiogenesis inhibitors, cell signaling modifiers, and gene therapy—all are active areas of research.
- Overcoming nitrosourea resistance with specific inhibitors.
- The prognostic effect of biologic markers and genetic aberrations.

## Pearls and Caveats

- Although the prognosis for these tumors generally is poor, there is a spectrum of survival possibilities for malignant glioma patients, particularly younger patients and those with anaplastic astrocytomas. Long-term survival occurs in a small percentage of patients. *Patients should be offered the choice to pursue aggressive therapies and thus the opportunity for long-term survival.*
- Elderly patients with large bilateral GBMs occasionally are palliated with a short course of radiotherapy such as 300cGy for 10 fractions.
- A single imaging modality, either CT or MRI, should be used serially to evaluate for response or progression.
- Distinguishing peritumoral edema from tumor radiographically is not reliable. Tumor cells have been identified histologically within the abnormal T2 signal area as well as in radiographically normal appearing brain.

## Suggested Reading

Berger MS, Wilson CB. *The Gliomas.* Philadelphia: W.B. Saunders, 1999.

DeAngelis LM, Burger PC, Green SB, Cairncross JG. Malignant glioma: Who benefits from adjuvant chemotherapy? *Ann Neurol.* 1998;44(4):691–695.

Kleihues P, Cavanee WK (eds). *Pathology and Genetics of Tumors of the Nervous System* (2nd ed). New York: Oxford University Press, 2000.

Levin VA. Chemotherapy for brain tumors of astrocytic and oligodendroglial lineage: The past decade and where we are heading. *Neuro-oncology.* 1999; 1(1):69–80.

Levin VA, Hoffman WF, Heilbron DC, Norman D. Prognostic significance of the pretreatment CT scan on time to progression for patients with malignant gliomas. *J Neurosurg.* 1980;52(5):642–647.

Moots PL. Pitfalls in the management of patients with malignant gliomas. *Semin Neurol.* 1998;18(2):257–265.

Shapiro WR. Therapy of adult malignant brain tumors: What have the clinical trials taught us? *Sem Oncol.* 1986;13(1):38–45.

Shapiro WR, Shapiro JR. Principles of brain tumor chemotherapy. *Sem Oncol.* 1986;13(1):56–69.

# 17

# Other Astrocytomas

Tumors of presumed or known astrocytic lineage other than the malignant astrocytomas are discussed here. This group includes a variety of tumors categorized by histology, location, age of onset, and natural history. Despite the common name *astrocytoma*, each of these tumors has a distinct biology, behavior, and pathogenesis. Most are tumors of childhood and young adulthood. Recognizing these tumors as distinct from the malignant gliomas is important because they tend to have a better prognosis and aggressive therapy is not always warranted. The term *low-grade glioma* is neither appropriate nor accurate, because it groups together several tumors with different behaviors, such as the pilocytic astrocytoma and the well-differentiated fibrillary astrocytoma. Furthermore, *low grade* tends to be misinterpreted by both physicians and patients as equivalent to *benign*. In general, these astrocytoma variants proliferate very slowly and patients require long-term follow-up. Unfortunately, survival at 10 years does not necessarily represent a cure.

## Well-Differentiated Astrocytoma

The well-differentiated astrocytoma, or grade II astrocytoma (WHO classification), is a diffuse, infiltrating central nervous system (CNS) tumor, with a median age at diagnosis of 30 years. Although slower growing and histologically less aggressive than the malignant astrocytomas, these generally are incurable with current therapies. Furthermore, many ultimately progress to become malignant astrocytomas. Patients typically present with seizures, headaches, or neurologic deficits.

Radiologically these tumors are hypodense on nonenhanced computed tomography (CT) images or hypointense on T1 magnetic resonance imaging (MRI) sequences and do not enhance with contrast agents. CT scans can be normal. T2 MRI sequences reveal bright signal in involved areas. Histologically, cellularity is increased compared with normal brain, and astrocyte nuclei may be enlarged. Necrosis, mitotic activity, and vascular changes are absent. Traditional approaches to these tumors have included either close observation or resection, depending on the patient's signs and symptoms and the tumor location. If resection can be performed, surgery should be the first step. Postoperative radiotherapy may benefit selected patients, particularly those with neurologic deficits and incompletely resected tumors. The timing of radiotherapy remains controversial. Historical series comparing immediate radiotherapy with observation are difficult to interpret because of the variation in treatments applied, patient selection criteria for treatment, and the retrospective nature of such studies. However, two large prospective trials have just been completed. The first evaluated two doses of radiotherapy and found them to be equivalent. Another trial randomized patients to immediate vs. delayed radiotherapy at clinical or radiographic progression. Immediate radiotherapy delayed progression but the overall outcome was similar.

## Ganglioglioma

These are histologically benign tumors, composed of a mixture of atypical neurons and astroctyes, and generally occur in children and young adults. Patients usually present with seizures. Typical locations include the temporal or frontal lobes, ventricles, and cerebellum. The radiographic appearance is that of a well-circumscribed low- or mixed-density lesion with minimal mass effect. Intra- or peritumoral cysts are common (40–50%), and these tumors occasionally erode the inner table of the skull. Maximal surgical resection generally is curative.

## Juvenile Pilocytic Astrocytoma

Juvenile pilocytic astrocytomas (JPA) typically are tumors of childhood and adolescence but can occur throughout the lifespan. Typical locations include the hypothalamus, optic pathways (optic chiasm, optic nerve, or both), thalamus, cerebellum, and cerebral hemispheres. The presentation depends on the size and location. Optic pathway tumors present with visual loss; they may be associated with neurofibromatosis type 1, especially when bilateral. Hypothalamic JPAs can cause precocious puberty. The radiographic appearance is that of a well demarcated and vividly enhancing mass. When associated with a cyst, the enhancing mass appears as a nodule along the wall of the cyst (mural nodule). Peritumoral edema is minimal, but mass effect is common. Complete surgical resection, when feasible, is curative. Certain locations, such as the optic pathways and hypothalamus, obviate complete surgical resection. Radiotherapy can slow progression. Malignant degeneration and seeding of the subarachnoid space are uncommon but do occur and may be transiently responsive to chemotherapy.

## Pleomorphic Xanthoastrocytoma

Pleomorphic xanthoastrocytomas (PXAs) are uncommon tumors that usually occur in the temporal or parietal cortex of adolescents and young adults. They present with seizures or symptoms related to mass effect. The histology is bizarre and may be misinterpreted as a glioblastoma. Most patients do well with surgical resection, although a subset of these tumors takes a more aggressive course and some recur as a glioblastoma.

## Dysembroplastic Neuroepithelial Tumor

Dysembroplastic neuroepithelial tumor (DNET) is a rare, cortically based neoplasm occurring from childhood to young adulthood. Usually patients have a long history of partial seizures; other symptoms are distinctly uncommon. Radiographically this tumor usually is nonenhancing and has the appearance of multiple small nodules. DNET often is confused with oligodendroglioma histologically. Calcification occurs but is much less common than in oligodendrogliomas.

## Subependymal Giant-Cell Astrocytoma

A distinct type of astrocytoma, subependymal giant-cell astrocytoma occurs almost exclusively in association with tuberous sclerosis. The tumors are located on the ependymal surface of the lateral ventricles and may cause ventricular obstruction. Symptomatic tumors or those causing obstructive hydrocephalus should be removed. Asymptomatic tumors do not require treatment. Malignant degeneration is rare.

## Suggested Reading

Berger MS, Wilson CB. *The Gliomas.* Philadelphia: W.B. Saunders, 1999.

Bigner DD, McLendon RE, and Bruner JM (eds). *Russell and Rubinstein's Pathology of Tumors of the Nervous System* (6th ed). New York: Oxford University Press, 1998.

Burger PC, Scheithauer BW. *Atlas of Tumor Pathology: Tumors of the Central Nervous System* (Third Series, Fascicle 10). Bethesda, MD: Armed Forces Institute of Pathology, 1993.

Kleihues P, Cavanee WK (eds). *Pathology and Genetics of Tumors of the Nervous System* (2nd ed). New York: Oxford University Press, 2000.

# 18

# Oligodendrogliomas

The oligodendrogliomas include low-grade oligodendroglioma, anaplastic oligodendroglioma, and oligoastrocytoma (mixed glioma). This group of tumors, although less common than astrocytomas, has received increased attention in the past decade because of reports of chemosensitivity and a favorable survival rate when compared with astrocytomas of similar grade. Nonetheless, the optimal therapy at diagnosis and recurrence remains undefined. Patients with oligodendrogliomas, particularly young patients with low-grade tumors, often enjoy a long period of tumor stability after initial diagnosis and treatment. Despite this indolent course, most patients ultimately die of tumor progression.

## Cell of Origin

Oligodendrogliomas originate from the oligodendrocyte, a myelin forming cell of the central nervous system (CNS).

## Median Age at Diagnosis

- Oligodendroglioma: 41 years.
- Anaplastic oligodendroglioma: 46 years.

## Incidence

- Oligodendroglioma: 0.29/100,000 person-years; 2.6% of intracranial tumors.
- Anaplastic oligodendroglioma: 0.07/100,000 person-years; 0.6% of intracranial tumors.

## Typical Locations

Supratentorial subcortical areas are the most frequent sites. Oligodendrogliomas rarely occur in the brain stem or spinal cord. Lesions usually are single, but multiple lesions have been reported, particularly in children. Intraventricular oligodendrogliomas must be distinguished from central neurocytomas, which are more common in that location.

## Presentation

Signs and symptoms of an intracranial lesion are discussed in Chapter 4. Seizures are the most common presenting feature (50% of patients) and occur during the course of the illness in most patients (88%).

## Radiographic Appearance

- Computed tomography (CT) scans show a well-demarcated hypodense subcortical mass. Calcification is common, and hemorrhage occurs in about 10% of tumors, including low-grade oligodendrogliomas. Enhancement is associated with anaplasia and is usually patchy.
- Magnetic resonance imaging (MRI) T1 images reveal a hypointense mass and T2 images show hyperintensity. The abnormal T2 signal represents both vasogenic edema and infiltrating tumor. Enhancement is associated with anaplastic oligodendrogliomas and is irregular and patchy. Ring enhancement is uncommon and is associated with a poorer prognosis.

## Pathology

Grossly, oligodendrogliomas appear as well-circumscribed, gray-pink masses. Cystic changes, necrosis, calcification, and hemorrhage often are apparent grossly or microscopically. Microscopically, there is a uniform appearance of closely packed swollen cells. The nuclei stain darkly and are surrounded by a clear halo ("fried-egg" appearance). The simplest and most commonly used grading system is that of "oligodendroglioma" and "anaplastic oligodendroglioma." Other systems using three or four tiers also are in use but provide no additional prognostic information.

## Nervous System Staging

Obtain a detailed neurologic history and examination. At presentation, a cranial MRI suffices. Second lesions within the nervous system are uncommon but occur more often than with astroctyomas. However, leptomeningeal spread may occur with tumor progression; and if patients develop spinal symptoms, an enhanced spinal MRI is warranted.

## Systemic Staging

Systemic metastases are rare and tend to occur only in patients who have survived several years and have anaplastic tumors. The most common locations are lung, liver, and bone. Systemic symptoms more often are due to unrelated medical problems or systemic complications of treatment. Systemic symptoms should be evaluated as clinically indicated.

## Usual Treatment

- Because of the significant potential toxicity associated with available therapies for oligodendrogliomas and the tumor's indolent natural history, treatment must be individualized, based on tumor location, tumor grade, patient symptoms, and other comorbidities.
- *Surgery* provides a diagnosis, may relieve symptoms, and prolongs survival.
- As with astrocytomas, maximal resection, while preserving neurologic function, improves survival.
- Anaplastic oligodendrogliomas require immediate treatment. Historically, *radiotherapy* has been used postoperatively. This approach clearly delays recurrence and prolongs survival.
- As with low-grade astrocytomas, the optimal timing of radiotherapy for low-grade oligodendrogliomas is unclear. Radiotherapy has been recommended for symptomatic or incompletely resected tumors. However, radiotherapy may be deferred in neurologically normal patients whose seizures are well controlled by anticonvulsant agents until there is clinical or radiographic progression. The disease can be indolent for years and the neurotoxic effects of radiotherapy must be considered.
- A radiation dose of 60 Gy is appropriate for anaplastic tumors, but only 54 Gy is needed for low-grade oligodendrogliomas.
- The role of *chemotherapy* for low-grade oligodendrogliomas is evolving, and some form of chemotherapy ultimately may replace radiotherapy as initial treatment for both oligodendrogliomas and anaplastic oligodendrogliomas. PCV (procarbazine, CCNU, vincristine) is the chemotherapy regimen best studied for low-grade and anaplastic oligodendrogliomas and causes measurable tumor regression in 75% of patients. Platinum-containing regimens, temozolamide, and melphalan are active second-line agents.

## Outcome

The median survival for low-grade oligodendroglioma patients may exceed 10 years. Anaplastic oligodendroglioma patients have a median survival of 5–7 years. The same prognostic factors that are important for malignant astrocytomas are important for oligodendrogliomas. However, in practice, it is impossible to predict outcome for individual patients.

## Areas of Investigation

- Sequencing chemotherapy before radiotherapy, dose intensification, radiosensitizers, and non-nitrosourea-based chemotherapy regimens—all are active areas of research.
- Correlation of chemotherapeutic response and prognosis with genetic abnormalities, such as p53 mutations and 1p and 19q deletions.
- Improving the diagnostic accuracy of oligodendroglioma vs. astrocytoma.

## Suggested Reading

Glass J, Hochberg FH, Gruber ML, et al. The treatment of oligodendrogliomas and mixed oligodendroglioma-astrocytomas with PCV chemotherapy. *J Neurosurg.* 1992;76(5):741–745.

Levin VA. Chemotherapy for brain tumors of astrocytic and oligodendroglial lineage: The past decade and where we are heading. *Neuro-oncology.* 1999; 1(1):69–80.

Mason WP, Krol GS, DeAngelis LM. Low-grade oligodendroglioma responds to chemotherapy. *Neurology.* 1996;46(1):203–207.

Paleologos NA, Cairncross GJ. Treatment of oligodendroglioma: An update. *Neuro-oncology.* 1999;1:61–68.

# 19

# Brain Stem Gliomas

Brain stem glioma is a distinct category of central nervous system (CNS) tumor because of its unique location and behavior. These are unresectable tumors by virtue of their location. The histology of brain stem gliomas spans the spectrum of gliomas located elsewhere in the CNS. Therapeutic approaches parallel treatments for malignant gliomas but are less rewarding. Although 80% of brain stem gliomas occur in childhood, there is a second peak in early adulthood and cases occasionally occur in older patients.

## Typical Locations and Presentation

There are three distinct types of brain stem gliomas, although overlap can occur. It is helpful to consider these distinct types because signs and symptoms depend on the region of the brain stem involved. Furthermore, the natural history and approach to therapy is determined by the tumor location.

### Pontine Gliomas

The pons is the primary site of involvement in 80% of brain stem gliomas. Most patients present with cranial nerve (CN) involvement (especially CN VI and VII), upper motor neuron signs, and ataxia. Hydrocephalus is uncommon at diagnosis. Children also may present with irritability, change in personality, or change in sleep pattern.

### Tectal Gliomas

This type of brain stem glioma has been recognized with the advent of modern neuroimaging. A subset of patients with idiopathic aqueductal stenosis based on computed tomography (CT) scans have tectal gliomas when examined with magnetic resonance imaging (MRI). These patients present with hydrocephalus and occasionally Parinaud's syndrome or other abnormalities of extraocular movements.

### *Exophytic Cervicomedullary Lesions*

Patients with exophytic cervicomedullary lesions typically have an extended history of vomiting or headaches. Focal neurologic deficits are less common, but lower cranial nerve deficits, particularly dysphagia or drooling, are typical.

## Radiographic Appearance

MRI is the imaging procedure used to diagnose and follow patients with brain stem gliomas. These lesions can be missed on CT scans.

- In pontine glioma, diffuse enlargement of the pons is best appreciated on saggital images. The lesion appears hypointense or isointense on T1 images and hyperintense on T2. Enhancement is variable and can be patchy, ring-like, or absent. The appearance of new enhancement in the absence of a change in overall size is of uncertain significance but probably represents dedifferentation.
- Tectal gliomas usually are limited to the dorsal midbrain but may involve nearby structures. The lesions typically are hyperintense on T2 images and usually do not enhance.
- Cervicomedullary junction gliomas appear as exophytic masses that are isointense to hypointense on T1 images, hyperintense on T2 images, and have vivid and homogenous enhancement (similar to pilocytic astrocytomas). Cyst formation may occur.

## Pathology

The pathology of brain stem gliomas can range from a low-grade astrocytoma to a glioblastoma. Oligodendrogliomas are rare. Enhancement on MRI does not necessarily indicate a malignant tumor. Dorsal exophytic tumors can be biopsied fairly easily, but tumors completely intrinsic to the brain stem usually are diagnosed by MRI alone.

## Nervous System Staging

No nervous system staging is required. Neurofibromatosis should be considered.

## Systemic Staging

Systemic metastases do not occur. Systemic symptoms are due to unrelated medical problems or systemic complications of treatment.

## Usual Treatments and Outcome

### Pontine Gliomas

- The prognosis for pontine glioma is poor with any of the available therapies. Association with NF 1 may predict a more indolent course.
- Extensive resection is not possible, given the location of the tumor. The risk of neurologic deterioration is significant and histologic diagnosis does not predict outcome or dictate therapy. Therefore, surgery is avoided.
- Radiotherapy is the most frequently used treatment and results in temporary alleviation of signs and symptoms in most patients. Doses typically range from 5500 to 6000 cGy. With this approach, 80% of patients die within 18 months. Some adults can have a more protracted and benign course.
- A variety of chemotherapeutic agents have been tested for brain stem gliomas but none prolong survival. Chemotherapy sometimes is given to young children to control progression and defer radiotherapy.

### Tectal Gliomas

- Most patients remain stable for months to years following initial diagnosis. Cerebrospinal fluid (CSF) diversion relieves symptoms if hydrocephalus is present. Radiotherapy is not advocated at initial diagnosis. Careful follow-up is indicated.
- There is limited information regarding treatment for patients whose tumors progress. Radiotherapy probably is helpful.

### Exophytic Cervicomedullary Lesions

- Extensive resection for many patients is possible, and some are stabilized for months to years with this approach.
- Since most are low-grade gliomas, the benefit of radiotherapy is unclear.

## Pearls and Caveats

- The interpretation of historical series and clinical trials for brain stem gliomas is difficult, because many patients were treated before the availability of MRI, most patients were not biopsied, and all types of brain stem glioma have been included together.

- Although the diagnosis of brain stem glioma usually is correct, the clinician should be aware of alternative diagnoses that may mimic brain stem glioma either clinically or radiographically. These include brain stem encephalitis (viral or autoimmune), brain stem encephalopathies (disorders of mitochondrial enzymes), vascular malformations, and multiple sclerosis. Appropriate diagnostic testing, including repeat MRI scanning and CSF examination, should be performed as indicated.

## Suggested Reading

Landolfi JC, Thaler HT, DeAngelis LM. Adult brainstem gliomas. *Neurology.* 1998;51(4):1136–1139.

Packer RJ. Brain stem gliomas: Therapeutic options at time of recurrence. *Pediatr Neurosurg.* 1996;24(4):211–216.

Packer RJ, Nicholson HS, Johnson DL, Vezina LG. Dilemmas in the management of childhood brain tumors: Brain stem gliomas. *Pediatr Neurosurg.* 1991–1992;17(1):37–43.

Shiminski-Maher T. Brainstem tumors in childhood: Preparing patients and families for long- and short-term care. *Pediatr Neurosurg.* 1996;24(5): 267–271.

# 20

# Pituitary Region Tumors

A wide variety of tumors can occur in and around the sella tur-
cica. The most common tumors in this region are craniopharyn-
giomas, pituitary adenomas, meningiomas, and optic chiasm
gliomas. Visual impairment is a common presenting symptom,
due to compression or invasion of the optic chiasm. Hormone-
related symptoms also are common, due to compression or involvement of the pituitary gland or hypothalamus. Although
most tumors in this region are histologically benign, their proximity to the optic chiasm, carotid arteries, and cavernous sinus
can result in significant disability.

## Clinical Presentations

Tumors of the sella and suprasellar region typically present
with either visual or hormone-related symptoms. Figure 20-1 illustrates the
anatomy of the sella, cavernous sinus, optic chiasm, and other adjacent structures. The most common visual deficit is a bitemporal hemianopsia (Figure
20-2), which is due to compression of the optic chiasm. Other atypical visual
field deficits also occur. Endocrinologic symptoms relate to either compression of the pituitary gland and subsequent hypopituitarism or overproduction
of a pituitary hormone by a pituitary adenoma. Patients also develop hypopituitarism as a result of treatments, such as radiotherapy. Refer to standard
medical texts for further details regarding endocrinologic evaluations.

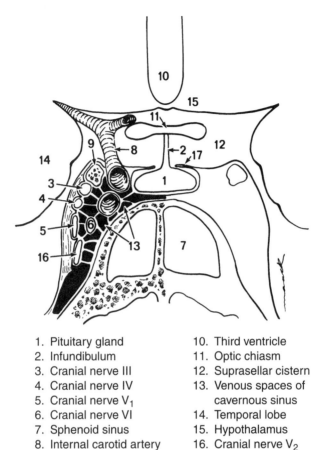

1. Pituitary gland
2. Infundibulum
3. Cranial nerve III
4. Cranial nerve IV
5. Cranial nerve V$_1$
6. Cranial nerve VI
7. Sphenoid sinus
8. Internal carotid artery
9. Anterior clinoid process
10. Third ventricle
11. Optic chiasm
12. Suprasellar cistern
13. Venous spaces of cavernous sinus
14. Temporal lobe
15. Hypothalamus
16. Cranial nerve V$_2$
17. Diaphragma sellae

**Figure 20-1**  Anatomy of the sella and parasellar region. (Reprinted with permission from Osborn AG. *Handbook of Neuroradiology.* St. Louis: Mosby, 1991:332.)

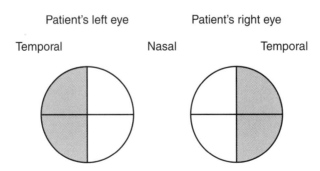

**Figure 20-2**  Bitemporal hemianopsia. Note that the visual field deficit may be incomplete.

## Differential Diagnosis of Sellar and Parasellar Mass Lesions

The most common entities are

- Pituitary microadenoma (<1.0 cm).
- Pituitary macroadenoma (>1.0 cm).
- Optic chiasm glioma (see Chapter 24).
- Meningioma (see Chapter 23).
- Craniopharyngioma.
- Carotid aneurysm.
- Arachnoid cyst.
- Metastasis (see Chapter 28).
- Lymphocytic hypophysitis.

### Craniopharyngioma

#### Incidence

The incidence of craniopharyngioma (CP) is 0.11/100,000 person-years, and it represents 0.9% of intracranial tumors.

#### Presentation

CP typically is a tumor of children, adolescents, and young adults. Symptoms arise due to compression of the optic chiasm, the pituitary gland, and the third ventricle. Therefore, visual field deficits, hormonal aberrations including diabetes insipidus, and symptoms of hydrocephalus are common. Children may present with obesity and other growth abnormalities including precocious or delayed puberty.

#### Radiologic Features

- Lesions are located both intrasellar and suprasellar (70%), suprasellar only (20%), and intrasellar only (10%).
- Calcification is common.
- Computed tomography (CT) scans reveal a heterogeneous solid or cystic mass. Enhancement is heterogeneous.
- Magnetic resonance imaging (MRI) scans reveal a heterogeneous mass. Portions are isointense to hyperintense on T1 and hyperintense on T2. Enhancement of solid masses or a cyst rim is seen.

#### Pathology

Grossly, these are encapsulated, solid, or cystic tumors. Microscopically, there are sheets of epithelial cells arranged in layers, keratinized cells, connective tissue, cholesterol crystals, and areas of lamellar bone.

**Treatment and Outcome**

The primary treatment for CP is resection via a frontal craniotomy, transphenoidal approach, or combined procedure. Although these are benign tumors, they often are quite large and extend into neighboring structures. Therefore, surgical removal can be challenging and some tumors cannot be resected completely. Endocrinologic sequelae including panhypopituitarism and diabetes insipidus are common. When gross-total resection is not accomplished, postoperative radiotherapy is administered and associated with a decrease in progression. Long-term follow-up is warranted.

## Pituitary Adenoma

### Incidence

Pituitary adenomas (PAs) are the most common tumors of the pituitary region. Many PAs are subclinical, as evidenced by the frequency with which they are found incidentally at autopsy. Symptomatic PAs occur in <1% of the population but about 10% of people are found to harbor a PA at autopsy.

**Presentation**

For microadenomas,

- Symptoms can result from overproduction of an anterior pituitary hormone.
- Hyperprolactinemia causes galactorrhea and amenorrhea in females and hypogonadism in males (52% of PAs).
- Excessive growth hormone causes gigantism and acromegaly (27% of PAs).
- Adrenocorticotropic hormone (ACTH) secreting tumors cause Cushing's syndrome (20% of PAs).
- Thyroid-stimulating hormone (TSH) secreting tumors, causing hyperthyroidism, are rare.

For macroadenomas,

- Pituitary insufficiency is due to compression of the pituitary gland or stalk.
- Mild hyperprolactinemia is due to disruption of the pituitary stalk and loss of inhibition from the hypothalamus.
- Visual field deficits are due to compression of optic chiasm (bitemporal hemianopsia).
- Oculomotor paresis results from cavernous sinus involvement.
- Headaches relate to traction on the diaphragmata sella.

### Radiologic Features

- Microadenomas are visualized as masses of <1.0 cm that are low density on CT scans within the brightly enhancing normal pituitary gland. Calcification is rare.
- Macroadenomas typically are isodense on CT scans and enhance uniformly. If hemorrhage is present, the lesion is hyperdense before contrast. On MRI scans, these tumors are isointense on T1 and slightly hyperintense on T2. Enhancement is uniform. If hemorrhage is present, the signal characteristics are mixed. Calcification occurs more often than with microadenomas.

### Treatment

Pituitary adenomas are managed medically or surgically, depending on the patient's symptoms, tumor size, and secretory status. Hormone inhibition usually is the first approach and effective in most patients. When this approach fails, transsphenoidal removal of the tumor using microsurgical techniques usually is successful in reversing endocrine aberrations. Larger tumors or those causing optic chiasm compression are managed surgically with the goal of decompressing the optic chiasm. Gross total removal usually is not possible, and the residual tumor is stabilized with radiotherapy. Radiotherapy is more effective in controlling tumor growth than in reversing hypersecretory syndromes. Serial formal visual field examinations are important in following these tumors.

## Suggested Reading

DeVita VT, Hellman S, Rosenberg SA. *Cancer: Principles and Practice of Oncology.* Philadelphia: Lippincott-Raven, 1997.

McCord MW, Buatti JM, Fennell EM, et al. Radiotherapy for pituitary adenoma: Long-term outcome and sequelae. *Int J Radiat Oncol Biol Phys.* 1997;39(2):437–444.

Osborn AG. *Handbook of Neuroradiology.* St. Louis: Mosby, 1991.

Rush S, Cooper PR. Symptom resolution, tumor control, and side effects following postoperative radiotherapy for pituitary macroadenomas. *Int J Radiat Oncol Biol Phys.* 1997;37(5):1031–1034.

# 21

# Germ Cell and Pineal Region Tumors

Most tumors of the pineal region are either germinomas or pineal cell tumors, and are tumors of adolescents and young adults. Presentation relates to the location in the nervous system rather than histology. Accurate tissue diagnosis is essential for planning therapy and can be achieved with low morbidity with modern surgical techniques. In selected cases, noninvasive diagnosis is achieved by cerebrospinal fluid (CSF) tumor markers or cytology. Overall, 5-year survival rates range from 44% to 90% and vary with the type of tumor, age, extent of disease at diagnosis, and therapy.

## Types of Pineal Region Tumors

- Germ cell tumors.
- Pineal tumors (pinealomas and pineoblastomas).
- Meningiomas.
- Lymphomas.
- Gliomas.
- Metastatic tumors.
- Pineal cysts.

## Presentation

The classic presentation of a pineal region mass is Parinaud's syndrome: paralysis of conjugate upward gaze, light-near pupillary dissociation, and retraction convergence nystagmus. With the advent of magnetic resonance imaging (MRI) scanning, most pineal tumors are diagnosed and treated before quadraparesis occurs. Other clinical features may include headache, nausea or vomiting, lethargy, ataxia, and diplopia. Germ cell tumors can also involve the suprasellar region and present with endocrine aberrations, including growth abnormalities (obesity), pituitary insufficiency (hypothyroidism, adrenal insufficiency), and diabetes insipidus.

## General Approach and Diagnosis

CSF diversion is indicated to alleviate hydrocephalus. Until recently, the pineal region was difficult to approach surgically and patients were treated with CSF diversion and empiric radiotherapy. However, with the advent of modern surgical techniques, particularly microsurgery and ventriculoscopy, tissue diagnosis and gross total resection often are feasible. For germ cell tumors and pineoblastomas, staging of the neuraxis with MRI and CSF examination is essential. These studies should be done preoperatively or deferred for 10–14 days postoperatively to avoid diagnostic confusion related to the presence of surgical debris in the CSF. The CSF is examined for cytology and the tumor markers alpha-fetoprotein (AFP, in yolk sac tumors), human chorionic gonadotropin (B-HCG, in choriocarcinoma), and human placental alkaline phosphatase (hpALP, in germ cell tumors).

## Germ Cell Tumors

### Classification

- Germinoma (pure germinomas arise from germ cells, multipotent embryonal cells).
- Nongerminomatous germ cell tumors:
  – Endodermal sinus tumor (yolk sac tumors)
  – Choriocarcinoma
  – Teratoma (benign, mature teratoma and malignant, poorly differentiated teratoma).

### Age and Gender Distribution

The age of onset generally is 12–40 years. Pineal germ cell tumors occur primarily in men, suprasellar germ cell tumors occur primarily in women.

### Incidence

About half of pineal region tumors are germ cell tumors, with an incidence of 0.09/100,000 person-years. They represent 0.6% of intracranial tumors.

## Typical Locations

Typically, these tumors are located in the pineal (60–80%) or suprasellar (20–30%) region. Germ cell tumors, particularly nongerminomatous germ cell tumors, spread along CSF pathways and about 10% are multifocal at diagnosis and may involve the pineal gland, hypothalamus, walls of the third ventricle, or leptomeninges.

## Radiographic Appearance

- Germ cell tumors are well-delineated pineal or suprasellar masses that usually are hyperdense on noncontrast computed tomography (CT) scans. Calcification is common (50–70%) and most cases show strong, homogeneous enhancement. On MRI scans, germ cell tumors appear isointense on T1 and isointense to hyperintense on T2. Enhancement is intense and often heterogeneous. CSF pathway metastases are identified with contrast-enhanced MRI scans.
- Teratomas tend to have mixed signal characteristics, including fat, cysts, calcification, and hemorrhage.
- Despite these generalizations, neuroimaging findings are nonspecific and do not correlate reliably with histologic findings.

## Staging

All patients should have enhanced cranial and spinal MRI scans at diagnosis. Both CSF and serum should be studied for tumor markers (AFP, B-HCG, hpALP).

## Pathology

Germinomas are histologically identical to testicular seminomas and ovarian dysgerminomas. Two distinct cell populations are seen: Large polygonal or spheroidal cells with vacuolated cytoplasm and large round nuclei are mixed with normal appearing lymphocytes. Germinomas stain for placental alkaline phosphatase, which occasionally can be measured in the CSF.

## Treatment and Outcome

- Risk factors for recurrence of germ cell tumors include multifocality, positive CSF cytology, positive CSF tumor markers (B-HCG or AFP, but not hpALP), and the presence of embryonal elements other than mature teratoma.

- Radiotherapy:
  - Most pure germinomas are cured with radiotherapy.
  - Focal germinomas without poor risk factors usually are treated with regional radiotherapy (pineal and ventricular system).
  - Patients with evidence of neuraxis dissemination are given craniospinal radiation.
- Chemotherapy: Preirradiation chemotherapy, particularly for patients at higher risk, has been studied with the goal of increasing the cure rate.
  - Only preliminary data are available documenting the safety of reducing radiation dose for pure germinomas and controlled data on preirradiation chemotherapy are lacking.
  - When chemotherapy is used alone for germ cell tumors, relapses requiring radiotherapy occur in 50% of patients within 2 years. This is true for both germinomas and nongerminomatous germ cell tumors.
  - Preirradiation chemotherapy is used for patients with malignant germ cell tumors (nongerminomatous germ cell tumors). Active agents include cisplatin, bleomycin, cyclophosphamide, and vincristine. Chemotherapy generally is given for 3–6 courses, after which patients are restaged. Patients with localized tumors then receive focal radiation therapy and patients with disseminated tumors receive craniospinal irradiation with boosts to the ventricular system and pineal region.

## Pinealomas

### Classification

- Pineocytoma (benign tumor of pineal cells).
- Pineoblastoma (primitive neuroectodermal tumor, PNET).

### Mean Age at Onset

- Pineocytomas: adolescence to mid-life.
- Pineoblastomas: childhood to adolescence, occasionally young adults.

### Typical Locations

Although the typical location is the pineal gland, pineoblastomas also spread along CSF pathways.

### Radiographic Appearance

- Pineocytomas appear isodense or hyperdense on CT scans and enhancement usually is prominent. Calcification is common. On MRI scans, they have variable signal intensity.

- Pineoblastomas are isodense to hyperdense on CT scans with vivid enhancement. On MRI scans, they are isointense to hypointense on T1, isointense to hyperintense on T2, and enhance vividly. Calcification is uncommon.
- In general, pineocytomas are smaller than pineoblastomas at diagnosis.
- Recurrent pineoblastomas may not enhance.

## Pathology

Pineocytomas are slow-growing neoplasms that microscopically appear similar to the normal pineal gland. Pineoblastomas are hypercellular neoplasms composed of small, poorly differentiated cells and microscopically resemble medulloblastomas and other PNETs.

## Treatment and Outcome

With modern surgical techniques, pineocytomas often can be removed completely, and no further therapy is indicated unless the disease recurs. Although pineoblastomas can be removed surgically, adjuvant chemotherapy and radiation are recommended analogous to therapy for medulloblastomas (see Chapter 22). Multiagent chemotherapy is given, followed by neuraxis radiotherapy.

## Suggested Reading

Robertson PL, DaRosso RC, Allen JC. Improved prognosis of intracranial non-germinoma germ cell tumors with multimodality therapy. *J Neurooncol.* 1997;32(1):71–80.

Schild SE, Haddock MG, Scheithauer BW, et al. Nongerminomatous germ cell tumors of the brain. *Int J Radiat Oncol Biol Phys.* 1996;36(3):557–563.

Schild SE, Scheithauer BW, Haddock MG, et al. Histologically confirmed pineal tumors and other germ cell tumors of the brain. *Cancer.* 1996; 78(12):2564–2571.

# 22

# Medulloblastoma and Other Primitive Neuroectodermal Tumors

Medulloblastoma and other primitive neuroectodermal tumors (PNETs) are a group of highly aggressive central nervous system (CNS) tumors with a tendency to spread via cerebrospinal fluid (CSF) pathways. These typically are tumors of childhood and young adulthood. PNETs are both radiosensitive and chemosensitive, and outcomes with aggressive therapy may lead to prolonged survival in some patients. Medulloblastoma, the most common PNET of the CNS, is reviewed here.

## Terminology, Pathology, and Classification

Because tumors in a variety of locals have an identical histologic appearance, they have been classified under the general term *primitive neuroectodermal tumors*. PNETs are embryonal tumors originating from primitive neuroepithelial cells. Histologically, they are hypercellular, homogeneous tumors composed of small cells that stain blue with hemotoxylin and eosin. Cells are arranged in dense sheets and often form rosettes. PNETs are related to other small, blue-cell tumors outside the CNS, such as small-cell lung cancer, Ewing's sarcoma, and Wilms' tumor. However, in the nervous system, the location of these tumors has a major prognostic impact. Their biologic behavior and outcome varies greatly; these are not equivalent neoplasms that just happen to occur in different parts of the CNS. For example, medulloblastoma is curable in 60% of patients, whereas long-term survival with pineoblastoma or central neuroblastoma is rare. A better understanding

114

and classification of these tumors will likely await molecular characterization.

Types and locations of CNS PNET include

- Medulloblastoma: cerebellum.
- Pineoblastoma: pineal gland (see Chapter 21).
- Retinoblastoma: retina.
- Neuroblastoma: cerebral hemispheres.
- "Trilateral tumor": bilateral retinoblastomas and pineoblastoma.

## Medulloblastoma

### Age at Onset

Most medulloblastomas occur in childhood, with 50–60% occurring during the first decade. A lesser peak occurs between ages 20 and 30 years.

### Incidence

Medulloblastoma accounts for roughly one third of CNS tumors in children.

### Typical Locations

Medulloblastomas typically occur in the cerebellar vermis in children and the cerebellar hemisphere in adolescents and young adults. Spread via CSF pathways is common, with 20–30% of patients presenting with CSF metastases. Systemic metastasis, primarily to the long bones, occurs in about 5% of patients.

### Presentation

Young children with medially located medulloblastomas present with symptoms of increased intracranial pressure (ICP), including headache, nausea or vomiting, and somnolence. Truncal ataxia also is common. Older children and young adults with laterally located tumors tend to present with ataxia, followed by symptoms of increased ICP as the tumor grows. Subarachnoid spread often is subclinical.

### Radiographic Appearance

- Complete imaging of the neuroaxis (brain and spinal cord) is indicated at diagnosis.
- Cysts, hemorrhage, and calcification are common.

- Computed tomography (CT) scans reveal a hyperdense mass with homogeneous and vivid enhancement.
- On magnetic resonance imaging (MRI) scans, medulloblastomas are isointense or hypointense on T1, hyperintense on T2, and enhancement typically is vivid and homogenous. Enhancement is absent in some patients, especially after treatment.

### Nervous System Staging

MRI scans of the brain and entire spine and CSF examination for cytology are necessary in all patients and important for planning treatment. Spine MRI scans and lumbar puncture should be performed either preoperatively or 2–3 weeks after definitive surgical resection to eliminate misdiagnosis from postoperative debris.

### Systemic Staging

Many physicians perform a bone scan at diagnosis, but the yield is very low in asymptomatic patients. Bone marrow biopsy is unnecessary. Other symptoms should be evaluated accordingly.

### Usual Treatment and Outcome

The prognosis for medulloblastoma patients relates to the extent of disease at diagnosis. Poor risk factors include postoperative residual tumor of >1.5 cm, brain stem invasion, CSF pathway metastasis (by MRI or CSF examination), metastasis to the cerebrum, and age <3 years. Following radiotherapy alone, the incidence of 5-year disease-free survival of good and poor risk patients is 60–70% and 25–30%, respectively.

- Surgery:
  - Posterior fossa craniotomy for aggressive resection improves prognosis.
  - CSF diversion typically is postponed until resection is completed, as resection obviates the need for shunt in many patients.
  - A ventriculoperitoneal shunt is needed in about 30% of patients.
- Radiotherapy:
  - Medulloblastoma is one of the most radiosensitive tumors of the CNS.
  - Craniospinal irradiation (35 Gy) is given at diagnosis with a boost (55 Gy) to the posterior fossa.
- Chemotherapy:
  - Multiple agents are active in medulloblastoma, including the platinums, etoposides, cyclophosphamide, and nitrosoureas.

– Historically, chemotherapy has been used at relapse or for tumors resistant to radiotherapy.
– Chemotherapy plus radiotherapy substantially improves survival of poor risk patients and has become the current standard of care.
– The potential benefit of adding chemotherapy to radiotherapy in standard risk patients is under study.

### Recurrence

Typical sites of recurrent disease include

• Posterior fossa (50%).
• Frontal lobes (20%) and cerebrum.
• Bone (10–15%): long bones and ribs.
• Suprasellar region.

## Suggested Reading

Cohen BH, Packer RJ. Chemotherapy for medulloblastomas and primitive neuroectodermal tumors. *J Neurooncol.* 1996;29(1):55–68.

David KM, Casey AT, Hayward RD, et al. Medulloblastoma: Is the 5-year survival rate improving? A review of 80 cases from a single institution. *J Neurosurg.* 1997;86(1):13–21.

Jenkin D. The radiation treatment of medulloblastoma. *J Neurooncol.* 1996; 29(1):45–54.

Rorke LB, Trojanowski JQ, Lee VM, et al. Primitive neuroectodermal tumors of the central nervous system. *Brain Pathology.* 1997;7(2):765–784.

Zeltzer PM, Boyett JM, Finlay JL, et al. Metastasis stage, adjuvant treatment, and residual tumor are prognostic factors for medulloblastoma in children: Conclusions from the Children's Cancer Group 921 randomized phase III study. *J Clin Oncol.* 1999;17(3):832–845.

# 23

# Meningiomas and Other Meningeal Tumors

Meningioma is the most common tumor in the central nervous system (CNS). Although most are slow growing and histologically benign, they can induce significant symptoms depending on location. Complete surgical resection is curative in about 80% of patients. When resection is not complete, roughly 40% of cases recur within 5 years of surgery. Radiotherapy can cause tumor stabilization in many patients with recurrent disease. Hormonal manipulation and cytotoxic chemotherapy have been disappointing. Up to 10% of meningiomas are malignant, and they carry a less favorable prognosis. Other meningeal-based tumors are described briefly.

## Benign Meningioma

### Mean Age at Onset

The mean age at onset is 62 years.

### Incidence

The incidence is 2.63/100,000 person-years. These represent 25% of intracranial tumors and 25% of intraspinal tumors.

### Gender Distribution

- Intracranial meningiomas: female/male ratio is about 2:1.
- Spinal meningiomas: female/male ratio is about 9:1.

## Cell of Origin

These tumors originate in arachnoidal cells.

## Typical Locations

- Meningiomas usually are single but can be multiple, especially in familial syndromes or when associated with neurofibromatosis type 2.
- Parasagittal or convexity tumors represent 30–40% of meningiomas.
- Sphenoid wing tumors represent 15–20% of meningiomas.
- Olfactory groove or planum sphenoidale tumors represent 10% of meningiomas.
- Suprasellar tumors represent 10% of meningiomas.
- Falcine tumors represent 5% of meningiomas.
- Meningiomas can occur anywhere there is meningeal tissue, including the cavernous sinus, clivus, foramen magnum, trigone of the lateral ventricles, optic nerve sheath, and sites of ectopic meninges.
- Spinal meningiomas most often are thoracic and tend to occur laterally.

## Presentation

The presentation of a meningioma depends on its location. Meningiomas can grow to an extensive size if located in clinically "silent" areas of the brain, such as the frontal lobes. Since they are dural based and slow growing, patients commonly present with seizures or headaches. Base of the skull meningiomas present when they are smaller, and they are one cause of skull-base syndromes (see Chapter 34).

## Radiographic Appearance

- Computed tomography (CT) scans show a homogeneously enhancing, dural-based lesion with a "dural tail." Minimal to extensive peritumoral edema is present. Of meningiomas, 15–20% are calcified. Hyperostosis of adjacent bone may be present. Hemorrhage is rare.
- Magnetic resonance imaging (MRI) scans are isointense to gray matter on most sequences, hyperintense on T2; if calcified, areas of hypointensity show up on T2. The appearance of meningioma on CT and MRI scans is similar, but MRI can better define the relation to vascular structures, identify dural sinus occlusion, and may reveal a second lesion not visualized on CT scans.
- Rare cases of nonenhancing meningiomas have been reported.
- The differential diagnosis of meningioma includes extramedullary hematopoiesis, dural metastasis, CNS sarcoid, and chloroma.

## Pathology

Grossly, meningiomas are well circumscribed and arise from the dura mater. Benign meningiomas do not invade brain parenchyma. Some meningiomas grow *en plaque* along the dura mater and can be very extensive. Microscopically, meningiomas can form one of several patterns (e.g., endotheliomatous, fibroblastic). These patterns are of no particular prognostic importance except for secretory meningiomas, which are associated with significant edema, and papillary meningiomas, which are biologically aggressive.

## Nervous System Staging

MRI of brain. MRI of spine as indicated by signs and symptoms, or if the patient has neurofibromatosis type 2. Patients with meningiomas in proximity to the optic nerve should be examined by an ophthalmologist prior to surgery or other interventions.

## Systemic Staging

No systemic staging is required.

## Usual Treatment and Outcome

- Some meningiomas can be followed carefully and require no immediate treatment.
- Surgical resection: Survival for meningioma patients has improved significantly as a result of modern surgical methods. When resection is complete, only 20% of patients suffer recurrences. However, when surgical resection is incomplete, approximately 40% of patients develop symptomatic recurrence within 5 years.
- Radiotherapy: Conformal radiotherapy can stabilize tumors for patients with unresectable or recurrent meningiomas. The role of single-fraction radiosurgery for benign meningiomas is being defined but is limited to lesions ≤3 cm. Stereotactic radiotherapy (focused fractionated therapy) is appropriate in selected cases to minimize risks to nearby structures.
- Hormonal therapy: Hormonal therapy is of theoretical interest because meningiomas can enlarge with pregnancy. Estrogen and progesterone receptors are present in 20–40% and 80% of tumors, respectively. Estrogen receptor blockage with tamoxifen has caused antecdotal tumor stabilization; however, such reports should be interpreted with caution because of the known intermittent growth pattern of meningiomas. Progesterone receptor blockage with mifepristone is of no clear benefit.

- Chemotherapy: Cytotoxic therapy with hydroxyurea has been reported anecdotally to slow meningioma growth; larger trials are in progress with hydroxyurea as well as temozolamide.

### Areas of Investigation

Areas of investigation include hormonal manipulation, cytotoxic chemotherapy, and interferon alpha-2B.

### Pearls and Caveats

Neither MRI nor CT scans can distinguish reliably a benign meningioma from an atypical or malignant meningioma or other meningeal-based tumor. If the decision is made to "observe" the lesion, initial scans should be done at short frequency (3–4 months) to determine growth pattern.

## Atypical and Malignant Meningiomas

Some meningiomas have more aggressive behavior. These are termed *atypical* (intermediate behavior) or *malignant* (most aggressive). In contrast to benign meningiomas, malignant meningiomas (MM) invade brain parenchyma, have a higher risk for recurrence, and may be more difficult to resect completely. Postoperative radiotherapy is recommended for patients with MM regardless of extent of resection. Response to radiotherapy is variable and many patients die of local recurrence. Five-year survival rates range from 41 to 85%.

## Hemangiopericytoma

Hemangiopericytoma (HPC) is an aggressive meningeal-based tumor previously classified as a meningioma (angioblastic meningioma) but now classified as a sarcoma under the World Health Organization classification of brain tumors. Resection should be followed by radiotherapy in all patients. Local recurrence and/or distant metastasis are common.

## Hemangioblastoma

Hemangioblastoma (HB) is an aggressive tumor that accounts for 1–2.5% of primary intracranial tumors. These tend to occur in young adult to middle-aged patients. HB tends to occur in the cerebellum. Of all hemangioblastomas, 10–20% occur in the context of von Hippel-Lindau (VHL) disease, in which case they tend to be multiple and involve the spinal cord and less commonly the cerebrum. Other features of VHL disease include retinal angiomas, renal cysts, renal carcinoma, pancreatic cysts, and pheochromocytoma. Treatment is surgical and radiotherapy is used for resistant or recurrent cases. HBs may be associated with polycythemia due to secretion of an erythropoietin-like factor.

## Suggested Reading

Glaholm J, Bloom HJ, Crow JH. The role of radiotherapy in the management of intracranial meningiomas: The Royal Marsden Hospital experience with 186 patients. *Int J Radiat Oncol Biol Phys.* 1990;8(4):755–761.

Kaba SE, DeMonte F, Bruner JM, et al. The treatment of recurrent, unresectable and malignant meningiomas with interferon alpha-2B. *Neurosurgery.* 1997;40(2):271–275.

Mahmood A, Caccamo DV, Tomecek FJ, Malik GM. Atypical and malignant meningiomas: A clinicopathological review. *Neurosurgery.* 1993;33(6):955–963.

Miralbell R, Linggood RM, de la Monte S, et al. The role of radiotherapy in the treatment of subtotally resected benign meningiomas. *J Neurooncol.* 1992;13(2):157–164.

# 24

# Tumors of the Optic Nerve and Chiasm

This chapter addresses the differentiation and management of tumors involving the orbit and optic pathways, which primarily include optic nerve gliomas and optic nerve sheath meningiomas. The goals for management are preservation of vision and tumor control.

## Orbital Masses

- Optic nerve meningioma.
- Optic nerve glioma.
- Optic neuritis.
- Metastatic tumors.
- Plexiform neurofibroma.
- Hemangioma.
- Schwannoma of the orbital branch of third nerve.
- Increased intracranial pressure or dilation of the subarachnoid space.

## Optic Nerve and Chiasm Gliomas

### Presentation

The presentation of optic nerve and chiasm gliomas depends on the location in the visual pathway.

- Intraorbital optic nerve glioma: monocular visual loss, strabismus, proptosis, and optic atrophy.
- Optic chiasm glioma: bitemporal hemianopsia, less specific visual field deficits.
- Hypothalamic glioma: developmental delay, ataxia, precocious puberty, weight loss, overactivity, euphoria.

## Epidemiology

- Gliomas of the optic nerve, chiasm, and hypothalamus account for 3% of primary brain tumors in children and 1% of adult gliomas.
- The most common tumor of the optic nerve/sheath complex is a glioma.
- Peak incidence is from ages 2 to 6 years.
- 10–20% of optic nerve/chiasm gliomas are associated with neurofibromatosis type 1. The percentage is higher when bilateral tumors are present.

## Radiographic Appearance

- Computed tomography (CT): fusiform low-density enlargement of the optic nerve, 50% enhance, calcification is rare.
- Magentic resonance imaging (MRI): isointense on T1, hyperintense on T2, 50% enhance. MRI is better for determining the extent of involvement and relation to other structures.

## Pathology

Most tumors of the optic pathways are pilocytic astrocytomas. Less common histologies include oligodendrogliomas or mixed gliomas, anaplastic astrocytoma, or glioblastoma.

## Treatments and Outcome

- Infant type: These present before one year of age, with large tumors invading the hypothalamus. In general, the prognosis is poor and early visual loss is common.
- Older children and young adult type: Older children and adults generally have tumors involving, in order of frequency, the optic nerve, chiasm, and hypothalamus. In general, vision is better preserved and the prognosis is somewhat better than in infants.
- The natural history of optic pathway gliomas is one of long periods of stability mixed with spurts of growth.
- Overall the 10-year survival is 60%.
- Surgery: Radical resection is indicated for those tumors with a large exophytic component or for cyst decompression, or, if complete visual loss has occurred, surgery is then with curative intent.
- Radiotherapy: Radiotherapy is given for optic nerve and chiasmal gliomas when there is unequivocal tumor progression. Tumors invading the hypothalamus usually require radiotherapy, although this is deferred in very young patients, if possible.

- Despite low-grade histology and slow growth rate, most patients experience progression of disease after radiotherapy.
- Treatment with radiotherapy can be associated with endocrine abnormalities and cognitive dysfunction.
- Chemotherapy: Aggressive regimens can delay the need for radiotherapy in young patients.

## Optic Nerve Meningiomas

### Background and Presentation

Optic nerve meningiomas arise from the meningeal sheath surrounding the optic nerve. They are histologically similar to meningiomas located elsewhere. The age of onset may be slightly younger than for intracranial meningiomas but generally later than for optic nerve gliomas. Symptoms include visual impairment, pain with eye movement, and orbital headaches.

### Radiographic Appearance

- CT: tubular involvement of the optic nerve sheath, strong enhancement around the nonenhancing optic nerve, calcification more common than for optic nerve gliomas.
- MRI: isointense enlargement of optic nerve sheath, enhancement around optic nerve.

### Pathology

See Chapter 23 for the pathology of meningiomas.

### Treatments and Outcome

The general approach to the treatment of meningiomas is outlined in Chapter 23. When meningiomas are confined to the orbit and visual loss is complete, resection is indicated and usually curative. For patients with partial visual impairment, preservation of vision is an important goal. Despite some risk of radiation optic neuropathy when optic nerve meningiomas are irradiated, the long-term risk of visual loss due to tumor progression is greater.

## Suggested Reading

Berger MS, Wilson CB. *The Gliomas*. Philadelphia: W.B. Saunders, 1999.

Garvey M, Packer RJ. An integrated approach to the treatment of chiasmatic-hypothalamic gliomas. *J Neurooncol*. 1996;28(2–3):167–183.

# 25

# Primary Central Nervous System Lymphoma

Primary central nervous system lymphoma (PCNSL), a rare central nervous system (CNS) tumor, occurs preferentially in immunocompromised patients; however, it is increasing in incidence in both the HIV and non-HIV populations. Nearly all are intermediate to high-grade B-cell lymphomas. Diffuse infiltration of the CNS is common and neuroimaging studies underestimate the extent of CNS involvement at diagnosis. Vitreous or cerebrospinal fluid (CSF) involvement occurs in 20% and 40% of patients, respectively, either at diagnosis or during the course of their illness. PCNSL is a tumor responsive to corticosteroids, chemotherapy, and radiotherapy. Unfortunately, such responses not always are durable and relapse is common. Preirradiation chemotherapy with a methotrexate-based regimen improves the chances of a durable remission.

## Cell of Origin

B-lymphocytes usually are the cell of origin.

## Mean Age at Onset

The mean age at onset is 54 years.

## Incidence

The incidence is 0.43/100,000 person-years. These represent 4.1% of intracranial tumors.

## Typical Locations

The typical locations of these tumors are the periventricular white matter, subcortical/cortical locations, leptomeninges, and vitreous. About 50% are single and 50% are multiple at diagnosis.

## Presentation

PCNSL presents with signs and symptoms typical of an intracranial mass lesion, as discussed in Chapter 4. A subset of patients presents with visual symptoms, such as "floaters," due to vitreous involvement. The response to corticosteroids usually is dramatic and may interfere with diagnosis if administered prior to biopsy.

## Diagnosis

The diagnosis of PCNSL usually is made by stereotactic biopsy, although occasionally CSF cytology or vitreous aspirate may establish the diagnosis. Corticosteroids should be withheld preoperatively because they may interfere with the diagnostic quality of the biopsy. Resection is not indicated because it does not improve the prognosis and may worsen the degree of neurologic deficit.

## Radiographic Appearance

### Non-HIV-Related PCNSL

- Computed tomography (CT)
  - Usually hyperdense on nonenhanced images, may be isodense.
  - Homogeneous enhancement is typical.
  - Calcification and hemorrhage are rare.
- Magnetic resonance imaging (MRI)
  - Isointense to hyperintense on T1 unenhanced images.
  - Hyperintense on T2 images.
  - Enhancement is homogeneous.
  - MRI is better for detection of small lesions and leptomeningeal involvement.

### HIV-Related PCNSL

- CT: Typically, there is ring-enhancement or patchy enhancement; occasionally, no enhancement is seen.
- MRI
  - As in the preceding, the tumor may not enhance.
  - Multiple bright nonenhancing areas are found in T2 images.

## Pathology

PCNSL appears histologically similar to systemic non-Hodgkin's lymphomas. Tumor growth tends to be perivascular, and the PCNSL may be infiltrated by reactive lymphocytes (T-cells).

## Nervous System Staging

Evaluation requires the following:

- Complete neurologic examination, including mental status.
- Cranial enhanced MRI scans, MRI with contrast of the spine if spinal signs or symptoms are present.
- Ophthalmologic evaluation with slit lamp examination to evaluate for vitreous involvement.
- Lumbar puncture for cytology, cell counts, protein, and glucose.

## Systemic Staging

- The incidence of systemic lymphoma at diagnosis of PCNSL is about 2–3%.
- If performed, only a chest X ray and CT of the abdomen and pelvis are necessary. Bone marrow biopsy is extremely low yield.

## Treatment and Outcome

- Radiotherapy: Postoperative radiotherapy results in high response rates and improved survival over supportive therapy. Response durations are short and the median survival with radiotherapy alone is 10–18 months.
- Chemotherapy: Methotrexate-based chemotherapy followed by whole brain radiotherapy then high-dose cytarabine was associated with a high response rate, a median survival of 40 months, and a 5-year survival of 22.3% in a single institution series. Many of the patients treated in this manner developed cognitive dysfunction or ataxia, particularly those over age 60.
- Preliminary results using a similar regimen in a cooperative group study have been reported (DeAngelis, 1999).
- Encouraging preliminary results have been reported in older patients treated with chemotherapy alone. The median survival was 33 months without cognitive impairment (Abrey, 2000).
- Osmotic blood/brain barrier enhanced, methotrexate-based chemo-therapy in a single institution series resulted in a median survival of 40.7 months with no demonstrable cognitive injury following 1 year of

treatment. This approach is extremely expensive, invasive, and a multi-institution trial has not been performed.

## Areas of Investigation

The following areas of treatment await future investigation:

- Conventional chemotherapy alone.
- Induction chemotherapy followed by high-dose chemotherapy with autologous stem cell rescue.
- Reduced radiotherapy dose in patients with complete response after chemotherapy.
- Osmotic blood/brain barrier disruption-enhanced chemotherapy delivery multicenter randomized trial.

## References

Abrey LE, Yahalom J, DeAngelis LM. Treatment for primary CNS lymphoma: The next step. *J Clin Oncol.* 2000;18(17):3144–3150.

DeAngelis LM, Seiferheld W, Schold SC, et al. Combined modality treatment of primary central nervous system lymphomas (PCNSL): RTOG 93-10. *Proceedings ASCO.* 1999;18:140a (abstract).

## Suggested Reading

Abrey LE, DeAngelis LM, Yahalom J. Long-term survival in primary CNS lymphoma. *J Clin Oncol.* 1998;16(3):859–863.

Blay J-Y, Conroy T, Chevreau C, et al. High-dose methotrexate for the treatment of primary cerebral lymphomas: Analysis of survival and late neurologic toxicity in a retrospective series. *J Clin Oncol.* 1998;16(3):864–871.

Freilich RJ, DeAngelis LM. Primary central nervous system lymphoma. *Neurol Clin.* 1995;13(4):901–914.

McAllister LD, Doolittle ND, Guastadisegni PE, et al. Cognitive outcomes and long-term follow-up after enhanced chemotherapy delivery for primary CNS lymphoma. *Neurosurgery.* 2000;46(1):51–60.

# 26

# Primary Spinal Cord Tumors

Primary spinal cord tumors are uncommon and most are either astrocytomas or ependymomas.

### Epidemiology

The incidence of primary spinal cord gliomas for males is 0.14/100,000 per person-year and for females 0.11/100,000 per person-year. Ependymomas account for 54% of primary spinal cord tumors, and their peak incidence is in the third to sixth decades. Astrocytomas account for 40% of primary spinal cord tumors and typically occur in children and young adults.

### Locations

- Astrocytomas occur primarily in the cervical and upper thoracic spinal cord and usually extend over several spinal segments.
- Ependymomas tend to occur in the lower thoracic and lumbar regions and also may extend over several segments.
- A distinct form of ependymoma, the myxopapillary ependymoma, occurs in the conus and filum terminale.

### Presentation

The presentation of spinal cord tumors is outlined in Chapter 5. Most patients present with progressive pain and myelopathy. Some patients have symptoms for several months to years prior to diagnosis. Myxopapillary ependymomas, which tend to be hemorrhagic, can present with acute subarachnoid hemorrhage or chronic hemorrhage producing meningeal siderosis. However, they usually present with back pain and radicular symptoms.

## Radiographic Appearance

Spinal cord tumors are best imaged with magnetic resonance imaging (MRI).

- *Spinal astrocytomas* appear as areas of spinal cord enlargement and are isointense to the spinal cord on T1 and hyperintense on T2. Areas of previous hemorrhage appear as decreased signal on T1 or T2. Enhancement is patchy and irregular.
- *Spinal ependymomas* are isointense to the spinal cord on T1 and hyperintense on T2. Hemorrhage has a characteristic hypointense rim on T1 and T2 images. Enhancement is intense and sharply demarcated.
- Multiple sclerosis plaques (inflammatory lesions) can mimic intradural tumor both radiographically and clinically.

## Treatments and Outcome

- Surgery: The aggressiveness of surgery depends on the type of lesion. Complete resection for ependymomas can be curative, and so aggressive resection usually is warranted. Astrocytomas are infiltrative and complete resection rarely is possible.
- Radiotherapy:
  - Postoperative radiotherapy is used for astrocytomas.
  - Radiotherapy is used for recurrent and progressive ependymomas but is not given following initial gross total resection of myxopapillary lesions.
- Chemotherapy: Chemotherapy for spinal cord astrocytomas parallels treatment for intracranial tumors. Carboplatin has stabilized tumors for some patients with spinal ependymomas at recurrence.

## Suggested Reading

Berger MS, Wilson CB. *The Gliomas.* Philadelphia: W.B. Saunders, 1999.
Schold SC Jr, Burger PC, Mendelsohn DB, et al. *Primary Tumors of the Brain and Spinal Cord.* Boston: Butterworth–Heinemann, 1997.

# 27

# Spinal Cord Metastasis

The management of spinal cord metastasis depends on whether or not the metastasis is causing epidural spinal cord compression as well as the overall status of the patient's systemic cancer. Important therapies include narcotic analgesics, corticosteroids, radiotherapy, and surgical intervention. Chemotherapy and hormonal therapies are employed in selected situations. Emergent treatment helps preserve or regain neurologic function. High-dose corticosteroid treatment and narcotic analgesics are valuable emergent therapy and always should be initiated during the evaluation for suspected spinal cord compression.

## Initial Management and Preventive Measures

Controlling pain is critical and should begin during the evaluation for spinal cord involvement with tumor. Patients with inadequate pain control have significant difficulties undergoing diagnostic testing. Furthermore, adequate pain control assists the patient in maintaining mobility and avoiding the complications of bedrest.

### Pain Control

- Narcotic analgesics and high-dose corticosteroids generally are required to adequately control pain.
- Some patients derive symptomatic benefit from wearing a brace or soft collar when out of bed.
- Prophylaxis for thromboembolic disease should be considered for patients who are not ambulatory.

- Bladder catheterization often is needed to avoid overflow incontinence, bladder discomfort, and obstructive nephropathy.
- A preventive bowel program, including stool softeners and rectal suppositories, is helpful for maintaining bowel function and preventing constipation and fecal impaction. Fecal retention due to spinal cord compression may be exacerbated by the use of narcotics and corticosteroids.

## High-Dose Corticosteroid Therapy

- High-dose corticosteroid therapy is effective in treating the pain associated with spinal cord metastasis and is associated with retained or regained neurologic function.
- Corticosteroids have lympholytic activity against lymphomas involving the epidural space.
- Corticosteroid therapy is a temporizing measure and needs to be followed by definitive treatment except in a palliative care setting.

## Specific Therapy

### Radiotherapy

Radiotherapy commonly is employed at some point following the diagnosis of epidural spinal cord compression. Radiotherapy usually improves pain control, lessens the need for analgesic agents, and can improve neurologic function. The smallest reasonable radiotherapy port is used to preserve bone marrow for future chemotherapy and limit side effects. However, evaluation of the entire spine prior to treatment planning is helpful in identifying other nearby areas of presymptomatic metastases. Failure of radiotherapy to improve symptoms may be due to bony compression of neural structures, unrelated nonmalignant processes (herniated disc), or progressive tumor. Recurrent neurologic symptoms following radiotherapy can be due to similar processes as well as subacute effects of radiotherapy on the spinal cord.

### Neurosurgical Intervention

Neurosurgical intervention remains a valuable management tool and should be considered when

- Radiotherapy fails to improve symptoms or neurologic deficits worsen following or during radiotherapy.
- There is spinal instability or compression by bony structures.
- There is no known primary tumor despite reasonable evaluation.
- The patient's tumor is known to be radio resistant.

- The diagnosis is unclear, such as suspected infection.
- Occasionally, as curative cancer surgery.

Careful selection of candidates for surgery is important. Potential risks and benefits should be considered for each patient. The risks of surgery in severely debilitated cancer patients are fairly high, whereas patients with good functional status may derive more benefit and be at lesser risk for complications. Operative candidates should be given prophylaxis for thromboembolic disease, as they are at significant risk.

In general, surgery is followed with radiotherapy as soon as possible, because the role of surgery is to relieve neurologic compromise rather than to remove the entire tumor.

### Hormonal Agents

Hormonal agents can contribute to the management of patients with hormone-sensitive tumors, such as breast cancer, but should not be expected to reverse major neurologic deficits. Tamoxifen may decrease the pain and minor neurologic symptoms associated with breast cancer metastasis.

### Chemotherapy

Chemotherapy generally is not used alone in the acute setting but could be considered in the asymptomatic or mildly affected patient (patients without myelopathy) and previously radiated patients who are not surgical candidates. Because the location of tumor generally is epidural, agents should be chosen based on their activity for the patient's tumor without regard to their ability to penetrate the central nervous system (CNS).

### Suggested Reading

Chamberlain MC, Kormanik PA. Epidural spinal cord compression: a single institution's retrospective experience. *Neuro-oncology.* 2000;1(2):120–123.

# 28

# Brain Metastasis

The occurrence of brain metastases represents a significant challenge in the care of patients with cancer. Symptoms may significantly alter the quality of life of affected patients, and brain metastases generally represent overall treatment failure. Long-term survival is poor. However, patients with central nervous system (CNS) metastasis can benefit from therapies that are either tumor specific or palliative, and specific therapy for some metastatic tumors can reduce symptoms and extend survival.

Three general situations exist for patients with metastatic brain tumors:

- *Brain metastases with no previous diagnosis of cancer and no apparent symptoms related to cancer.* A reasonable evaluation should take place in an effort to identify a primary tumor. However, this evaluation should not defer palliative or definitive cranial surgery. In general, a sufficient evaluation includes a complete physical examination, chest X ray, and computed tomography (CT) scans of the chest, abdomen, and pelvis. Based on the extent of systemic disease, location of the intracranial tumor, and other factors, resection of single brain metastasis is reasonable. Surgical intervention also is warranted if evaluation does not disclose a primary tumor amenable to tissue diagnosis.
- *Brain metastases present concurrently with other evidence of systemic tumor.* Treatment for this clinical presentation needs to be individualized and may include surgery if a single dominant or life-threatening brain metastases is present and chemotherapy may be used to combat certain chemoresponsive tumors.

- *Brain metastases develop in a patient with a known diagnosis of cancer.* Treatment also is individualized and depends on the patient's functional status, the number and location of brain metastases, and the extent of systemic disease.

No matter which of these clinical presentations is encountered, it is reasonable to direct treatment at the brain when this metastatic site is more likely to cause death or major disability than the systemic tumor or another metastatic site. This is the case roughly 50% of the time.

## Radiotherapy

A critical analysis of relevant randomized trials indicated that radiation therapy can effectively palliate the symptoms of brain metastases (Berk, 1995). Prognostic factors for improved quality of life and survival include good performance status and the absence of a non-CNS primary tumor (i.e., no systemic disease). The most efficient treatment protocol remains controversial but the literature supports the use of 20 Gy in five fractions for the treatment of patients with poor prognosis (Berk, 1995). Patients with a solitary brain metastasis and no evidence of systemic disease generally are best served by resection followed by postoperative radiation. Another reasonable approach includes whole brain irradiation followed by stereotactic radiosurgery, as appropriate. In cases of radioresistant tumors such as melanoma, single-fraction stereotactic radiosurgery without whole brain irradiation may be considered.

## Chemotherapy

Several regimens have demonstrated efficacy in patients with metastatic brain tumors from a variety of known primary sites or with an unknown primary tumor. One recent study includes a combination of thioguanine, procarbazine, dibromodulcitol, lomustine (CCNU), fluorouracil, and hydroxyurea (TPDC-FuHu) for progressive or recurrent metastatic tumors that failed to respond to surgery or radiation therapy (Kaba, 1997). Although toxicity is mild to moderate with this approach, the duration of response often is short. Other regimens have been employed with similar modest success. Temozolamide, a new and alkylating agent, is being evaluated in this setting.

## References

Berk L. An overview of radiotherapy trials for the treatment of brain metastases. *Oncology.* November 1995;9(11):1205–1212; discussion 1212–1216, 1219.
Kaba SE, Kyritsis AP, Hess K, et al. TPDC-FuHu chemotherapy for the treatment of recurrent metastatic brain tumors. *J Clin Oncol.* 1997;15(3):1063–1070.

## Suggested Reading

DeAngelis LM. Management of brain metastases. *Cancer Investigation.* 1994; 12(2):156–165.

Delattre J-Y, Krol G, Thaler HT, et al. Distribution of brain metastases. *Arch Neurol.* 1988;45:741–744.

Lang FF, Sawaya R. Surgical treatment of metastatic brain tumors [Review]. *Seminars in Surgical Oncology.* 1998;14(1):53–63.

Patchell RA. The treatment of brain metastases [Review]. *Cancer Investigation.* 1996;14(2):169–177.

Sawaya R, Ligon BL, Bindal AK, et al. Surgical treatment of metastatic brain tumors. *J Neuro-oncol.* 1996;27:269–277.

# 29

# Leptomeningeal Metastasis

Leptomeningeal metastasis (LM) is a rare complication of systemic cancer in which the leptomeninges are infiltrated by cancer cells. The overall incidence is 3–8% but is increasing as more cancer patients survive following initial treatment. With the exception of leukemia and lymphoma, the prognosis is poor and currently available therapies are considered palliative. Leptomeningeal dissemination also occurs in patients with primary brain tumors. Diagnosis of LM is important, because it affects overall management and, while rarely curative, therapy may provide significant palliation and extend survival for some patients. Timely diagnosis depends on a high index of clinical suspicion and vigorous diagnostic testing.

## Terminology

- General terms: *Leptomeningeal metastasis* is the most accurate term; other terms used synonymously include leptomeningeal disease, meningeal carcinomatosis, carcinomatous meningitis.
- In leukemia, *leukemic meningitis*.
- In lymphoma, *lymphomatous meningitis*.

## Sources of Metastasis

Metastasis can emanate from systemic cancers, such as

Breast cancer.
Small-cell lung cancer.
Non-small-cell lung cancer.
Acute leukemias.

Non-Hodgkin's lymphoma.
Melanoma.
Gastrointestinal cancers.

The primary tumor also may be located in the brain, as in

Malignant astrocytoma and oligodendrogliomas.
Medulloblastoma.
Pineoblastoma.
Germinoma.
Primary central nervous system lymphoma.

## Epidemiology

Overall, 3–8% of cancer patients develop LM. The incidence of LM is increasing, especially in breast and small-cell lung cancer patients and in HIV-related primary central nervous system lymphoma. Of patients surviving small-cell lung cancer for 3 years, 25% develop LM, and about 5% of breast cancer patients ultimately develop LM.

## Presentation

LM causes neurologic dysfunction at more than one level of the nervous system in a progressive, unremitting manner. With LM, 80% of patients have pain that is either spinal, radicular, meningeal, or a diffuse headache. Signs and symptoms can be divided into four groups:

- Brain: Symptoms include personality changes, cognitive impairment, labile affect, diminished alertness.
- Cranial nerves: Symptoms include one or more cranial neuropathies. Cranial nerve VII most commonly is affected.
- Spine: Symptoms include radiculopathy, myelopathy, sensory loss, reflex loss, urinary or fecal retention.
- Meningeal irritation: Seizures are the main symptom.

## Diagnosis

The major differential diagnosis in patients with suspected LM is multiple brain or epidural metastases and central nervous system (CNS) infection. In general, cranial nerves are affected earlier and to a greater extent in LM than infection. Fever and meningeal irritation in the setting of a normal neurologic exam suggest infection. Major parenchymal signs (hemiparesis, aphasia) are uncommon in LM and suggest brain metastases. The diagnosis of

LM is made by finding positive cerebrospinal fluid (CSF) cytology or diagnostic magnetic resonance imaging (MRI) findings in the appropriate clinical setting.

## Radiographic Appearance

- MRI scans are preferred over computed tomography (CT) scans.
- Diffuse leptomeningeal enhancement is seen on MRI scans. Small nodules may be present.
- Other conditions that cause diffuse meningeal enhancement include intracranial hypotension (post–lumbar puncture [LP]), infection, postcraniotomy, and recent head trauma, but none of these processes cause nodular enhancement.
- Communicating hydrocephalus.
- MRI scans can be normal in some patients.

## Nervous System Staging

Evaluation for suspected LM includes enhanced MRI scans of the brain and entire spine and CSF for cytology.

## Systemic Staging

In most cases of LM, the patient has known widespread systemic cancer. Despite this, patients generally die of their CNS disease. Investigations regarding the extent of systemic disease are directed by symptoms so that symptoms can be appropriately palliated.

## Treatment and Outcome

- Treatment for LM is usually palliative.
- Patients most likely to benefit from treatment are those with limited neurologic deficits, good performance status, absent or minimal parenchymal CNS metastases, and treatment-responsive systemic disease.
- Treatment should begin as soon as the diagnosis is confirmed.
- Radiotherapy: Radiotherapy is given to symptomatic areas and radiographically identified sites of bulky disease.
- Chemotherapy: Intrathecal chemotherapy provides palliation of neurologic symptoms in some patients.
  - Treatment through an Ommaya reservoir is preferred for ease of administration and better drug distribution in the CSF.
  - Methotrexate: The dosage is 12 mg two to three times a week; generally used for leukemias, lymphomas, and solid tumors.

- Cytarabine: The dosage is 40–50 mg two to three times a week; used primarily for leukemia and lymphoma. Liposomal cytarabine for intrathecal use also is available.
  - Thiotepa: The dosage is 10 mg two or three times a week.
- Systemic chemotherapy including high-dose IV methotrexate, cytarabine, and thiotepa has been used with success in some patients. Systemic toxicity is dose limiting.
- Patients with advanced disease and unreponsive primary tumors do not benefit from chemotherapeutic treatment of LM. Focal radiotherapy may palliate symptoms. The mean survival for these patients is about 6 weeks.
- The overall median survival for patients who are able to undergo therapy is less than 6 months. Meaningful palliation is provided in 50–90% of patients with reduced pain and improvement in neurologic deficits. A small subset of patients survives beyond a year.

## Suggested Reading

Balhuizen JC, Bots GT, Schaberg A, Bosman FT. Value of cerebrospinal fluid cytology for the diagnosis of malignancies of the central nervous system. *J Neurosurg.* 1978;48(5):747–753.

DeAngelis LM. Current diagnosis and treatment of leptomeningeal metastasis. *J Neurooncol.* 1998;38(2–3):245–252.

# VI

## Approach to
## Clinical Problems
## in Neuro-Oncology

# 30

## Anorexia and Weight Loss

Patients with advanced cancer report that anorexia, or loss of interest in food, is their second most common symptom after pain. The ability to eat is an important aspect of quality of life. This chapter focuses on the causes of anorexia and the weight loss that frequently accompanies this challenge to patient care. Included are strategies to improve appetite or adjust to lessened appetite.

### Causes of Anorexia in Cancer Patients

- Tumor related: The body may respond to the presence of a tumor by producing a number of endogenous substances, such as peptides, cytokines, and $\alpha_1$-glycoproteins. Furthermore, tumors can produce chemicals such as toxohormone-L.
- Patients may have cognitive deficits and/or fatigue that make meal preparation or eating a challenge.
- Treatment related: Anorexia can be a side effect of chemotherapy, radiation therapy, or medications for supportive care. Other gastrointestinal symptoms, such as nausea or vomiting, constipation, dysphagia, stomatitis, development of food aversions, and decreased sensation of taste and smell can be found simultaneously.
- Neurologic symptoms including dysphagia, apraxia, seizures.
- Oral candidiasis may cause taste alterations or pain when eating.
- Gastrointestinal difficulties may include treatment-related gastroparesis or constipation.
- Unrelated anorexia nervosa should also be considered, particularly in adolescent or young adult women.

- Depression. Because anorexia often increases a patient's feelings of depression, striving to improve appetite and minimize weight loss can enhance both physical and emotional well-being.

## Assessment of Anorexia

Key questions to ask in documenting potential causes and consequences of anorexia include the following:

- What were your favorite foods before your tumor diagnosis? Do you still like these foods? Is there anything that you especially want to eat now?
- What were your least favorite foods? Do you still dislike them?
- Has your sense of smell or taste changed?
- Is your mouth more sensitive to certain foods? If so, which ones?
- Are you having trouble swallowing?

The patient's medical records should contain sufficient information to document any weight loss that occurred concurrently with the onset of anorexia. If this information is unavailable, questions concerning "normal" (i.e., prior to tumor diagnosis) weight, recent weight loss, and changes in clothing fit may be asked. Remember, however, that a patient's statements about this matter may be a sensitive issue and may not be accurate. A family member or other individual close to the patient can corroborate the patient's responses or provide correct information.

## Suggestions for Managing Anorexia

- Have the patient eat several small meals per day, rather than three large meals at standard times.
- Figure out at what time of day attempts to eat are most successful, and plan a daily schedule so that a patient is able to eat at that time. Have food readily available so that the patient can eat whenever he or she is hungry.
- Because standard-sized food portions can be overwhelming, use smaller plates and beverage containers. Place small servings of several kinds of foods in muffin tins or other serving dishes with small compartments.
- Encourage the patient to eat what he or she chooses whenever feasible.
- Vitamins can be used to supplement dietary choices.
- High-calorie liquid food supplements in a variety of flavors are available in most large grocery stores and can be easy to drink and digest. However, these products can be costly and are not always appealing to patients. Patients often appreciate receiving samples to try before purchasing these products.

**Table 30-1**  Pharmacologic Agents That May Be Useful for Patients with Anorexia

| Agent | Dose Guidelines | Considerations |
|---|---|---|
| Corticosteroids | Dexamethasone: 2–4 mg qd<br>Prednisone: 10–20 mg qd | Also controls brain edema |
| Megestrol acetate | 40–160 mg bid | |
| Metoclopramide | 10–20 mg q 8 hours | Increases gastric emptying, improves gastroparesis |

- For the patient whose cognitive difficulties are interfering with food intake, a particular effort should be made to make mealtimes as enjoyable and social as possible. An added benefit of meals in a group setting is the assistance others can provide the patient in choosing nutritious foods and successfully completing a meal.
- Nutritionists and dieticians who specialize in working with cancer patients can provide valuable counseling and assistance.
- Positioning to provide optimal swallowing and prevent fatigue during mealtime.
- A number of pharmacologic interventions are available; these are listed in Table 30-1. In addition, ongoing clinical research is evaluating potential new agents in this arena.

## Suggested Reading

Bruera E, Fainsinger R. Clinical management of cachexia and anorexia. In D Doyle, GWC Hanks, N MacDonald (eds). *Oxford Textbook of Palliative Medicine.* Oxford, England: Oxford University Press, 1995.

Loprinzi CL, Kugler JW, Sloan JA, et al. Randomized comparison of megestrol acetate versus dexamethasone versus fluoxymesterone for the treatment of cancer anorexia/cachexia. *J Clin Oncol.* October 1999;17(10):3299–3306.

Waller A, Caroline NL. *Handbook of Palliative Care in Cancer* (2nd ed). Boston: Butterworth–Heinemann, 2000.

# 31

# Brain Tumors in Women of Childbearing Age

Women of childbearing age present special management issues related to the effects of various treatments on menstruation, fertility, and future childbearing. Women who are diagnosed with a brain tumor while pregnant or who become pregnant following their diagnosis face difficult choices and are in need of accurate information regarding their options. Management must be based on the patient's desires, stage of gestation, and nature of the tumor. Appropriate multispecialty care optimizes the chances for a positive outcome for both mother and baby.

## Brain Tumor Therapies and Menstruation, Fertility, and Childbearing Potential

- Tumors of the hypothalamus and pituitary region can cause infertility and amenorrhea.
- Brain irradiation can induce central hypogonadism due to injury to the pituitary and hypothalamus.
- Chemotherapy can cause temporary or permanent changes in menstruation and ovulation, particularly in patients over age 35. Menstrual periods can become irregular or cease altogether, causing premature menopause. Return of menses and fertility during or following chemotherapy can occur.
- Chemotherapy-induced infertility should not be assumed; reliable contraception should be used during treatment.
- The occurrence of mild to moderate thrombocytopenia during a menstrual period can increase blood loss due to menstruation. Severe

thrombocytopenia can be associated with life-threatening menstrual bleeding. If severe thrombocytopenia is anticipated with chemotherapy in a young woman, birth control pills can be used to control the menstrual cycle and assure contraception.

- Corticosteroids used to treat increased intracranial pressure (ICP) can decrease bone density over a period of months to years. Calcium and vitamin D supplementation should be considered (see Chapter 14).
- Anticonvulsant drugs, notably phenytoin, can cause osteoporosis.
- Return of normal menses following chemotherapy usually correlates with return of fertility.
- Women who do not resume normal menstrual periods within a few months following completion of treatment should be evaluated for hormone replacement therapy.
- There is no evidence that prior chemotherapy predisposes women to babies with birth defects. Oocytes are more likely to die from chemotherapy than mutate. However, there is an increased risk of low birth weight and spontaneous abortion following cancer therapy.

## Avoiding Pregnancy during Brain Tumor Therapy

- Avoiding pregnancy during brain tumor therapy is the safest course. Accurate information about contraception needs to be provided.
- A waiting period following the treatment of a brain tumor before considering pregnancy is sensible. This gives the woman an opportunity to begin recovering both physically and emotionally from the effects of treatment. A waiting period also allows the woman to make a decision based on the initial therapeutic results of treatment.

## Care of Pregnant Women with Brain Tumors

The presence of a brain tumor poses significant risks to both mother and unborn child. The mother faces all the serious medical and emotional challenges of any other brain tumor patient. In addition, she faces uncertainty regarding the effect of therapies on her unborn child, her own prognosis due to the brain tumor, and her own risks related to continuing or aborting the pregnancy.

### *Voluntary Termination of Pregnancy*

- Voluntary termination of pregnancy (abortion) depends on the stage of pregnancy. It is a personal decision for all women, with or without brain tumors, and is influenced by multiple cultural, political, financial, and religious factors. However, abortion is recommended for any woman with a malignant brain tumor in the first trimester of pregnancy.

- In areas where abortion is legal, the pregnant brain tumor patient may decide to have an abortion within the extent of the law. In most areas this is limited to the first trimester and early second trimester.
- For women in regions where abortion is illegal, a case for abortion may be made on medical grounds. Such an argument may be made if the tumor is inoperable, the patient has begun radiotherapy during the first trimester before pregnancy was diagnosed, first trimester chemotherapy was given or is deemed medically necessary, or if the maternal prognosis is very poor.
- In the third trimester, early induction of labor may be considered based on estimates of fetal viability.

## Imaging the Pregnant Woman

- Necessary neuroimaging should not be deferred because of pregnancy.
- Magnetic resonance imaging (MRI) scans are preferred over computed tomography (CT) scans during pregnancy to avoid fetal exposure to ionizing radiation. Gadolinium is avoided during the first trimester due to a lack of safety data.

## Maternal Risks

- Most of the risks associated with brain tumor in pregnancy are to the fetus.
- For the mother, the most concerning risk is that she will receive inadequate treatment for her tumor because of concern regarding effects of therapy on the unborn child.
- Pregnant women are not eligible for most clinical trials.
- Meningiomas and pituitary tumors can undergo accelerated growth during pregnancy.
- Pregnancy may worsen tumor-related symptoms due to hypervolemia and the effects of fatigue on pre-existing neurologic deficits.

## Fetal Risks

Fetal risks related to antitumor therapy include mutation, miscarriage, teratogenesis, birth defects, and cognitive abnormalities. Refer to Briggs, Freeman, and Yaffe's *Drugs in Pregnancy and Lactation* for comprehensive information regarding the risks of drug therapy during pregnancy and lactation. It must be emphasized that no chemotherapeutic agent is considered safe to the fetus.

## Corticosteroids

- As in nonpregnant patients, corticosteroids should be used at the lowest possible dose needed to control symptoms of increased ICP.
- There is no evidence that corticosteroids are teratogenic in humans.
- Exacerbation of pregnancy-related glucose intolerance can occur but generally is manageable.

## Surgery

- Lesions for which the optimal management is surgery should be managed accordingly.
- Craniotomy can be performed safely in pregnant women.
- Recent evidence suggests that the approach of postponing surgery until the time of fetal viability is not always the safest course. In fact, surgery later in pregnancy poses a significant risk of preterm labor because the uterus is more irritable.
- Decompression of an intracranial mass makes subsequent labor and delivery safer.

## Radiotherapy

- The risks of radiotherapy relate to the stage of gestation.
- The first trimester fetus is extremely sensitive to ionizing radiation, making the first trimester the period of highest risk. Even with abdominal shielding, maternal cranial irradiation exposes the fetus to ionizing radiation due to scatter. Doses as low as 2.5 Gy are associated with significant abnormalities when the exposure occurs between weeks 3 and 8.
- It is safest to wait until after delivery or abortion to perform radiotherapy. If this is not possible, radiotherapy should be deferred as far into the pregnancy as possible, at least beyond the first trimester, and then performed with abdominal shielding.

## Chemotherapy

- Risks to the unborn child from chemotherapy drugs also relate to the stage of gestation.
- Risks during the first trimester are greatest and include a high risk of spontaneous abortion and a high (17–40%) risk of major morphologic abnormalities.
- The risks are lower during the second and third trimesters and include low birth weight and granulocytopenia but not congenital anomalies. Nonetheless, chemotherapy is deferred until after delivery if possible.

**Table 31-1**    Guidelines for the Use of Antiepileptic Drugs during Pregnancy

1. Use first-choice drug for seizure type and epilepsy syndrome.

2. Use antiepileptic drug as monotherapy at the lowest dose and plasma level that protects against tonic-clonic seizures.

3. Avoid valproate and carbamazapine when a family history of neural-tube defects is present.

4. Avoid polytherapy, especially combination of valproate, carbamazepine, and phenobarbital.

5. Monitor plasma antiepileptic drug levels regularly and, if possible, monitor free or unbound plasma antiepileptic drug levels.

6. Continue folate daily supplement and ensure normal plasma and red cell folate levels during the period of organogenesis in the first trimester.

7. In cases of valproate treatment, avoid high plasma levels of valproate; divide doses over 3 or 4 administrations per day.

8. In cases of valproate or carbamazepine treatment, offer amniocentesis for alpha fetoprotein at 16 weeks and real-time ultrasonography at 18–19 weeks to look for neural tube defects; ultrasonography at 22–24 weeks can detect oral clefts and heart anomalies.

Source: Reproduced with permission from Delgado-Escueta and Janz, 1992.

## Labor and Delivery

- The presence of an intracranial mass lesion may increase the risks of vaginal delivery because of the possibility of cerebral herniation, particularly during the third stage of labor.
- Aggressive pain management during labor, including epidural anesthesia, helps control ICP by attenuating the bearing-down reflex.
- An intracranial mass lesion also may raise the risk of peripartum seizures and intratumoral hemorrhage.
- A third trimester MRI scan should be performed to provide updated information regarding the extent of mass effect prior to labor. If not performed or the patient's neurologic status has changed since it was done, a noncontrast CT scan should be considered during early labor. This should be done under fetal monitoring because prolonged supine positioning can compress the inferior vena cava and impair venous return to the heart, causing maternal hypotension and fetal distress.
- Cesarean section should be performed for the usual obstetrical reasons or for uncontrolled increased ICP.

## *Seizure Management*

The choice of anticonvulsant agents for the pregnant woman with epilepsy has been a controversial area of neurology. A consensus statement (Table 31-1) provides practical guidelines. Prophylactic anticonvulsant agents usually are not prescribed without a history of seizures.

## Suggested Reading

Allen HH, Nisker JA (eds). *Cancer in Pregnancy: Therapeutic Guidelines.* Mt. Kisco, NY: Futura Publishing, 1986.

Briggs GG, Freeman RK, Yaffe SH. *Drugs in Pregnancy and Lactation: A Reference Guide to Fetal and Neonatal Risk* (5th ed). Baltimore: Williams and Wilkins, 1998.

Cicuttini FM, Hurley SF, Forbes A, et al. Association of adult glioma with medical conditions, family and reproductive history. *Int J Cancer.* 1997; 71(2):203–207.

Delgado-Escueta AV, Janz D. Consensus guidelines: Preconception counseling, management, and care of the pregnant woman with epilepsy. *Neurology.* 1992;42(4 suppl 5):149–160.

Donaldson JO. *Neurology of Pregnancy* (2nd ed). Philadelphia: W.B. Saunders, 1989.

Isla A, Alvarez F, Gonzalez A, et al. Brain tumor and pregnancy. *Obstet and Gynecol.* 1997;89(1):19–23.

# 32

# Central Nervous System Infections

Central nervous system (CNS) infections are relatively uncommon in cancer patients but occur more frequently than in the general population and are more difficult to diagnose and treat. The spectrum of offending organisms also is different in immunocompromised patients than in the general population. Most CNS infections occur in patients with lymphoma and leukemia, and in patients recently treated with chemotherapy or corticosteroids. Signs and symptoms may be atypical compared with noncancer patients. Knowledge of the underlying tumor, associated immune deficits, and recent therapy guides diagnosis and initial empiric treatment.

## Meningitis

Meningitis occurs when infection involves the leptomeninges and may spread to the ventricular system.

### Presentation

- Acute bacterial meningitis typically presents with fever, nuchal rigidity, and headache over a period of hours to a few days.
- Signs and symptoms often are less typical and more indolent in cancer patients. Headaches may be masked by the opiate pain medications the patient already is taking, and fever may be minimal or absent.
- Nonbacterial meningitis presents with subacute symptoms, which initially may be subtle or nonspecific, including confusion, headache, photophobia, cranial nerve abnormalities, and fever.
- Cerebrospinal fluid (CSF) findings in meningitis are summarized in Table 32-1.

**Table 32-1**   CSF Findings in Meningitis

|  | *Bacterial* | *Viral* | *Fungal* | *Tuberculosis* |
|---|---|---|---|---|
| WBC/mm$^3$* | >200, mostly PMNs | 6–50, mostly lymphocytes | 50–200, mostly lymphocytes | 50–200, lymphocytes and polys |
| RBC/mm$^3$ | 5–10 | Herpes: 5–80 CMV: 0–5 | 0–5 | 0–5 |
| Protein (mg/dl) | >100 | 45–75 | >100 | >100 (up to 5000) |
| Glucose (mg/dl) | 20–45 (or <50% of blood glucose) | Usually normal | 20–45 (or <50% of blood glucose) | 20–45 (or <50% of blood glucose) |
| Other tests | Gram stain Culture Antigen tests | Serum and CSF viral titers PCR for viral DNA | Cryptococcal antigen, fungal cultures | AFB stain and culture |

WBC, white blood cell; RBC, red blood cell; PMNs, polymorphonuclear neutrophil leukocytes; CMV, cytomegalovirus; CSF, cerebrospinal fluid; PCR, polymerase chain reaction; AFB, acid fast bacilli.
*May be fewer WBCs early in the course or in patients with neutropenia.

## Sources

- Hematogenous (most common).
- Parameningeal structures (sinuses, middle ear, mastoid, vertebral bodies).
- Entry of organisms through defects in the skull or spinal column (uncommon but should be considered in patients with recent neurosurgical intervention, tumors invading the base of the skull, or trauma).
- Infection of implanted devices, such as ventriculoperitoneal shunts and Ommaya reservoirs.

## Organisms

- *Streptococcus pneumoniae, Neisseria meningitidis* (meningococcus), and *Haemophilus influenzae* are the most common organisms in immunocompetent patients.
- *Listeria monocytogenes* and *Cryptococcus neoformans* are the most common causes of meningitis in cancer patients and occur primarily in patients with lymphoma and leukemia.
  - *L. monocytogenes:*
    Anaerobic Gram positive rod (may falsely stain Gram negative).
    Organism is seen on Gram stain in only 10% of cases.
    Ampicillin is drug of choice, 500–1000 mg IV q 6 hours.

- *C. neoformans:*
  Onset of symptoms usually is slower than with *Listeria*.
  Predilection for basilar meninges.
  Cryptococcal antigen is positive in 80–95% of patients but in some patients it does not become positive for two or more weeks into the illness.
  Drug of choice is Amphotericin B. Consult a pharmacist regarding test dose and dose escalation.
  Fluconazole often is used in conjunction with Amphotericin B, 400 mg loading dose followed by 200–400 mg per day PO or IV.
  Fluconazole often is used for maintenance therapy, 100 mg per day PO or IV.
- In patients with neutrophil defects or neutropenia, meningitis usually is due to enteric Gram negative rods, such as *Pseudomonas* species and *Escherichia coli.*
- *Mycobacterium tuberculosis* causes a subacute to chronic meningitis with cranial nerve involvement and is uncommon in cancer patients.
- *Nocardia asteroides*
  - Branching Gram positive rod that is difficult to see on CSF Gram stain.
  - CNS involvement is present in up to half of patients with pulmonary infection.
  - Chorioretinitis is common.
  - Sulfadiazine is drug of choice, 2 g IV q 6 hours.
  - Shunt or reservoir infections usually is due to coagulase-negative *Staphylococcus* or skin organisms, such as *Proprionibacterium.*

## Brain Abscess

### Presentation

- The presentation of a brain abscess usually is nonspecific.
- Headaches (75%), nausea or vomiting (50%), seizures (33%), and neurologic deficits (<50%) are the most common presenting features.
- Papilledema (25%) and fever (10–20%) are present in a minority of patients and nuchal rigidity is absent unless there is associated meningitis.
- Radiologic findings are not specific. Abscesses may be single or multiple, hypodense (computed tomography, CT) or hypointense (magnetic resonance imaging, MRI), and demonstrate ring enhancement following contrast. During the early cerebritis stage, lesions may not enhance but are abnormal on T2 MRI scans. In general, the enhancing rim is thinner and more uniform than that seen with tumors or radiation necrosis.

- Needle biopsy usually is needed to identify the causative organism, and aspiration may improve symptoms by reducing the mass effect.

## Sources

- Oral flora.
- Sinuses.
- Enteric Gram negative rods.
- Pulmonary fungal infections.

## Organisms

*Toxoplasma gondii* and *Aspergillus* are the most common causes of brain abscess in cancer patients. *Nocardia* and *Candida* are less common causes. In chronically neutropenic patients, Gram negative rods and anaerobes are important causes.

- Toxoplasmosis
  - *Toxoplasma gondii* is a small obligate intracellular parasite that can be seen on Wright's or Giemsa stains.
  - Toxoplasmosis has a predilection for the basal ganglia and deep white matter of the cerebral hemispheres.
  - Toxoplasmosis also can manifest as meningoencephalitis.
  - Lesions usually are multiple.
  - Because toxoplasmosis is common, a therapeutic trial generally is recommended in suspected cases. Patients who do not respond or progress during therapy need to be biopsied.
  - Drug therapy includes sulfadiazine (25 mg/kg PO qid) and pyrimethamine (100 mg on day 1, then 50–75 mg PO per day); use folinic acid (5–10 mg PO qd) to minimize hematologic toxicty.
- Aspergillosis
  - Brain abscess is the most common manifestation of intracranial aspergillosis.
  - Aspergillosis is angioinvasive and can cause pseudoaneurysms (which can rupture) of large vessels at the base of skull. The abscesses can be hemmorhagic on CT or MRI scans.
  - Treatment is with Amphotericin B.

## Encephalitis and Meningoencephalitis

### Presentation

Encephalitis typically presents with seizures, mental status changes, asterixis, myoclonus, and occasionally focal neurologic deficits. Fever may or may not be present. Meningoencephalitis has a similar clinical picture, but signs and symptoms of meningeal irritation are more prominent. The cause of viral encephalitis in cancer patients usually is a virus of the herpes family but sporadic and seasonal forms (e.g., Western equine) also may occur.

### Varicella-Zoster Virus Encephalitis

Varicella-zoster virus (VZV) encephalitis occurs almost exclusively in immunocompromised patients. MRI scans typically reveal areas of increased signal on T2, which do not enhance, and are located in subcortical white matter (see the following).

### Cytomegalovirus encephalitis

- The features are typical of encephalitis, tropism for ventricular surfaces of lateral ventricles.
- Chorioretinitis is common.
- Diagnosis is by serum antibody titers and CSF study for polymerase chain reaction (PCR) detection of viral DNA particles.
- MRI scans show periventricular areas of T2 signal abnormality.

### Herpes Simplex Encephalitis

- This is a rare and potentially devastating CNS viral infection.
- The incidence may be increasing in the immunocompromised population.
- Typical clinical features include a change in behavior, memory and personality changes, seizures, headaches, and fever.
- The Herpes simplex virus (HSV) has a predilection for the temporal lobes and limbic structures. The frontal and parietal lobes also can be affected.
- On MRI scans, the areas of involvement are hypointense on T1, hyperintense on T2. Areas of hemorrhage are present in 50% of cases.
- Up to 50% of cases have bilateral abnormalities on MRI scans.
- Empiric treatment with IV acyclovir should be started as soon as the clinical suspicion of HSV encephalitis arises, 10 mg/kg IV q 8 hours. Follow with serum creatinine.
- Diagnosis is based on the clinical features, MRI findings, serum and CSF viral titers, and PCR for HSV.

### Progressive Multifocal Leukoencephalopathy

- Progressive multifocal leukoencephalopathy (PML) is an infection of oligodendrocytes with the JC virus and typically occurs in patients with lymphoma, chronic lymphocytic leukemia, or HIV disease.

- Patients present with features of encephalitis, including mental status changes, multifocal neurologic deficits, and cortical visual abnormalities but do not typically have headaches, seizures, or fever.
- CSF is normal on routine tests. The JC virus may be demonstrated with PCR.
- MRI shows multiple deep white matter abnormalities on T2 images that usually do not enhance and are not associated with mass effect.
- Biopsy can confirm the diagnosis but is not necessary if the CSF PCR is positive.
- There is no effective treatment for PML. There are anecdotal reports of responses to cytarabine and interleukin-2.

## Myelitis

*Myelitis* refers to infection of the parenchyma of the spinal cord, and it is usually viral. Infectious myelitis must be distinguished from the effects of chemotherapy, radiotherapy, and tumor, as discussed in Chapter 5. Both herpes simplex and varicella zoster can cause myelitis in immunocompromised patients. When due to the herpes viruses, the symptoms usually are preceded by a vesicular rash. The diagnosis is supported by PCR for viral DNA.

## Varicella-Zoster Virus

Varicella-zoster virus warrants further comment because it is a common viral infection in cancer patients, with many potential neurologic effects.

- Primary infection ("chicken pox"):
  - The primary infection with VZV tends to be more disseminated in the immunocompromised host than in the normal host.
  - Chicken pox can be complicated by Reye's syndrome if the patient is given aspirin-containing medications.
  - Acute ataxic meningoencephalitis presents with the onset of ataxia, nystagmus, and dysarthria, and usually follows the cutaneous rash by days to weeks.
- Cutaneous reactivation ("shingles") from the dorsal root ganglion with vesicular rash and neuropathic pain is the most common manifestation in adult cancer patients:
  - The incidence of postherpetic neuralgia is higher in cancer patients.
  - Dissemination beyond a single dermatome is more common in cancer patients.
  - Shingles may progress to myelitis in cancer patients.
  - Cerebral vasculitis and stroke can complicate facial zoster.

- Zoster myelitis presents within several days following the cutaneous rash. Occasionally the rash is absent. Weakness usually is asymmetric and may be one or more spinal levels below the rash.
- For zoster encephalitis see the previous discussion.

## Approach to the Patient with Suspected CNS Infection

- Cases of suspected meningitis are neurologic emergencies.
- Patients with other suspected CNS infections warrant urgent diagnosis and treatment.
- Initial empiric treatment is based on the suspected organisms and assumed immunologic defect related to the underlying tumor and recent therapies. Table 32-2 outlines an approach to empiric treatment based on these factors.
- The presence of systemic infection should be sought and may provide a diagnosis.
  - Perform a complete physical examination, in particular looking for Evidence of systemic infection, sinusitis, perirectal abscess. Rash with candidiasis, HSV, VZV, *Pseudomonas* sepsis, meningococcus. Retinitis seen with some fungal infections.
  - Blood cultures may provide culture diagnosis.
  - Chest X ray may disclose pulmonary infections such as *Nocardia* or *Aspergillus*.
- Lumbar puncture (LP) for CSF analysis should be performed in cases of suspected meningitis. If focal neurologic deficits or signs and symptoms of increased ICP are present, LP may be deferred until an imaging study is performed, but antibiotics should be started immediately.

## Pearls and Caveats

- Headaches may be mild and masked by narcotics the patient already is taking.
- Fever is less common than in nonimmunocompromised hosts.
- Nuchal rigidity uncommon, especially in neutropenic patients.
- Focal neurologic signs suggest involvement beyond the meninges, such as vasculitis, brain abscess, or encephalitis.
- CSF pleocytosis may be absent, especially in viral infections or neutropenic patients.
- The pneumococcal vaccine does not always prevent pneumococcal infection.
- If cranial nerve palsies are present, especially early in the course, suspect leptomeningeal involvement with tumor as an alternative diagnosis.

**Table 32-2**   Initial Treatment of Suspected CNS Infection in Cancer Patients, Based on Type of Immune Defect and Other Factors

| Immune Defect and Associated Causes | Common Causative Organisms | Initial Treatment and Diagnostic Tests |
|---|---|---|
| Neutropenia or neutrophil dysfunction<br>    Acute leukemia<br>    Some solid tumors<br>    Chemotherapy<br>    Corticosteroids | Gram negative rods<br>    *Pseudomonas*<br>      *aeruginosa*<br>    *Escherichia coli*<br>    *Klebsiella pneumoniae*<br>Gram positive rod<br>    *Listeria*<br>Gram positive cocci<br>    *Streptococcus*<br>    *Staphylococcus*<br>Fungi<br>    *Aspergillus* species<br>    *Candida* species<br>    Mucor | Ceftazidime and Gentamycin<br><br><br><br><br>Ampicillin<br><br>Vancomycin<br><br><br>Amphotericin |
| Splenectomy and B-cell abnormalities<br>    Hodgkin's disease<br>    CLL<br>    Hairy cell leukemia | *Streptococcus pneumoniae* | Cefuroxime and vancomycin |
| T-lymphocyte or mononuclear phagocyte defect<br>    Non-Hodgkin's<br>      lymphoma<br>    Hodgkin's disease<br>    CLL<br>    Steroids<br>    Some chemotherapy<br>      agents | *Listeria monocytogenes*<br>*Cryptococcus neoformans*<br>*Nocardia asteroides*<br>*Toxoplasma gondii* | Ampicillin<br>Amphotericin B<br>Amphotericin B<br>Sulfadiazine, pyrimethamine, and folinic acid |
| Immunoglobulin defects<br>    CLL<br>    Multiple myeloma<br>    Steroids | Herpes viruses: varicella zoster, cytomegalovirus, and herpes simplex | Acyclovir, gancyclovir<br>Cefuroxime or Nafcillin, consider Vancomycin for resistant pneumococci |
| Recent neurosurgical intervention or indwelling CNS catheter | *Staphylococcus aureus*<br>Coagulase-negative<br>    staphylococcus<br>*Proprionibacterium acnes* | Nafcillin (Vancomycin if MRSA* suspected), consider intrathecal therapy |

CLL, chronic lymphocytic leukemia.

*Methicillin-resistant *Staphylococcus aureus.*

- In up to 40% of cancer patients with both CNS and systemic infections, the CNS is infected by a different organism than the systemic organs.
- Involvement of cerebral blood vessels, particularly at the base of the skull, occurs with many CNS infections, especially aspergillosis. Resulting strokes are a cause of persistent neurologic deficits despite otherwise successful treatment of CNS infection.
- Since Hodgkin's disease rarely metastasizes to the brain, brain lesions in Hodgkin's patients are much more likely to be infectious than metastatic.

## Suggested Reading

Antunes NL, Hariharan S, DeAngelis LM. Brain abscesses in children with cancer. *Med & Ped Oncol.* 1998;31(1):19–21.

Brody MB, Moyer D. Varicella-zoster virus infection. The complex prevention-treatment picture. *Postgrad Med.* 1997;102(1):187–190, 192–194.

Galer BS, Portenoy RK. Acute herpetic and postherpetic neuralgia: Clinical features and management. *Mt Sinai J Med.* 1991;58(3):257–266.

Mandell GL, Douglas RG, and Bennett JE (eds). *Principles and Practice of Infectious Disease* (4th ed). New York: Churchill Livingstone, 1995.

Pruitt AA. Central nervous system infections in cancer patients. *Neurol Clin.* 1991;9(4):867–888.

Przepiorka D, Jaeckle KA, Birdwell RR, et al. Successful treatment of progressive multifocal leukoencephalopathy with low-dose interleukin-2. *Bone Marrow Transplan.* 1997;20(11):983–987.

Reusser P. Current concepts and challenges in the prevention and treatment of viral infections in immunocompromised cancer patients. *Supp Care in Cancer.* 1998;6(1):39–45.

Scheld WM, Whitley RJ, Durack DT. *Infections of the Central Nervous System.* New York: Lippincott-Raven, 1997.

Weaver S, Rosenblum MK, DeAngelis LM. Herpes varicella zoster encephalitis in immunocompromised patients. *Neurology.* 1999;52(1):193–195.

# 33

# Constipation

Constipation can be an uncomfortable and even debilitating problem that significantly reduces the patient's quality of life and may promote certain medical complications. This chapter discusses etiologies as well as options for prevention and treatment.

## Definition

Constipation is the difficult or infrequent passage of feces. Patients also may consider other gastrointestinal symptoms in their self-evaluation of constipation, specifically flatulence, bloating, tenesmus, nausea, and rectal pain.

## Contributing Factors

- Decreased activity level resulting from weakness, bed rest, routine of hospitalization, or habitual lack of adequate exercise.
- Nutritional factors, particularly inadequate fluid or fiber intake, and difficulty chewing so that food is not chewed well before swallowing and harder to digest.
- Change in food preferences, such as aversion to fruits and vegetables.
- Treatment-related factors, such as use of narcotic analgesics, tricyclic antidepressants, anticonvulsants; side effect of certain chemotherapeutic agents, such as vincristine and vinblastine; use of other drugs including corticosteroids.
- Unclean or otherwise unsatisfactory lavatory conditions; lack of privacy when using the lavatory.
- Tumor invasion of neural plexus or spinal cord compression.
- Medications, such as corticosteroids, certain chemotherapy agents, and narcotic analgesics.

## Assessment

Key questions to ask in documenting the causes and severity of constipation include the following:

- How is your bowel pattern different now, compared to what was normal for you before your tumor was diagnosed?
- How often have you taken laxatives in the past, and what have you taken?
- Are you now taking enemas, laxatives, suppositories, or other medications? (Some individuals have extensive previous history of chronic constipation or laxative dependence.)
- How often have you moved your bowels during the last five days? When was the last time you moved your bowels? Asking the patient or caregiver to write down a record of bowel movements can be useful. The actual frequency is not as important as associated symptoms such as bloating or hard, painful bowel movements.
- Are your bowel movements hard, soft, liquid? Bloody? Mucus containing?
- How much stool are you producing, compared to before tumor diagnosis?
- When you try to pass stool, do you have pain, cramps, or other discomfort?
- Do you feel as if you need to pass stool, but find yourself unable to do so?

## Examination

- Abdominal distention and tenderness.
- Bowel sounds.
- Fecal masses.
- Rectal examination: hard or impacted stool, an empty and dilated rectum (may be a sign of more proximal fecal impaction), hemorrhoids, fissures or fistulae.
- Hydration status.
- Consider plain films of the abdomen if history or physical examination suggests obstruction or ileus.

## Prevention

The patient who receives treatment known to cause constipation should be put on a prophylactic bowel program that includes the following:

- Maximizing dietary fiber or institution of fiber supplements.
- Stool softeners or laxatives, with specific guidelines provided regarding frequency of use.
- Enemas or digital stimulation, especially in patients with spinal cord tumors.

- Adequate fluid intake.
- Assess lavatory arrangements and suggest changes as feasible. Use of a bedside commode, if possible, often is preferable to a bedpan.
- Preventive measures are especially important before treatments known to cause neutropenia, as enemas and digital stimulation are avoided during neutropenic episodes.
- Adequate exercise may become a low priority once cancer is diagnosed. Encouraging regular light exercise whenever possible may help with constipation-related problems. Cancer patient support groups and other organizations may provide opportunities for walking and other exercise options.

## Treatment

- Many of the suggestions for prevention can be instituted once constipation has become a problem.
- The necessity of constipating medications should be reassessed.
- Mild laxatives: milk of magnesia, docusate sodium.
- Stronger laxatives: magnesium citrate, lactulose.
- Rectal suppositories.
- Enemas.

## Suggested Reading

Sykes N. Constipation and diarrhoea. In D Doyle, GWC Hanks, N MacDonald (eds). *Oxford Textbook of Palliative Medicine.* Oxford, England: Oxford University Press, 1995.

Waller A, Caroline NL. *Handbook of Palliative Care in Cancer* (2nd ed). Boston: Butterworth–Heinemann, 2000.

# 34

# Cranial Nerve Syndromes

The cranial nerves (CN) can be affected directly by primary or metastatic brain tumors. Cranial neuropathies also can result from chemotherapy, radiation, or central nervous system (CNS) infections. Knowledge of the normal anatomy of the CN and their surrounding structures is essential for evaluating cranial neuropathies in cancer patients. Unrelated neurologic diseases such as multiple sclerosis can cause CN symptoms. This chapter provides an approach to evaluation of cranial neuropathies.

### Anatomy and Function

Table 34-1 lists the cranial nerves, their anatomy, functions, and the pathologies that occur in cancer patients. Careful physical examination of the CN combined with the patient's history narrows the differential diagnosis and directs imaging studies.

### Pathogenesis

The more common cranial neuropathies and their causes are considered here.

#### Chemotherapy Agents

- Cisplatin can cause tinnitus, hearing loss, and vestibulopathy (CN VIII).
- Vincristine can cause optic atrophy, ptosis, CN VI, VII, VIII, IX, or X dysfunction.
- Tamoxifen can cause macular edema with blurred vision and rarely causes a true retinopathy.

**Table 34-1** Cranial Nerves, Skull Foramina, Function, and Pathology

| Cranial Nerve | Skull Foramina or Fissure (Other Structures Present) | Symptoms | Differential Diagnosis |
|---|---|---|---|
| I. Olfactory | Cribiform plate of ethmoid bone (ethmoidal arteries) | Loss of smell | Chemotherapy agents<br>Tumor<br>Surgery<br>Radiotherapy |
| II. Optic | Optic canal (oph-thalamic artery, dura and subarach-noid space) | Decreased visual acuity | Chemotherapy agents<br>Radiotherapy<br>Sellar masses<br>Metastases |
| III. Oculomotor | Superior orbital fis-sure (superior oph-thalmic vein and CN IV, $V_1$, VI) | Diplopia<br>Horner's syndrome<br>Superior orbital fis-sure syndrome | Direct involvement by tumor at cavernous sinus, superior orbital fissure, or Gas-serian ganglion |
| IV. Trochlear | Superior orbital fis-sure (superior oph-thalmic vein and CN III, $V_1$, VI) | Diplopia<br>Superior orbital fissure syndrome | Direct involvement by tumor |
| $V_1$ Trigeminal<br><br>$V_2$<br><br>$V_3$ | Superior orbital fis-sure (superior oph-thalmic vein and CN III, IV, VI)<br>Foramen rotundum (also inferior orbi-tal fissure)<br>Foramen ovale | Facial numbness<br>Weakness of mus-cles of mastication | Infection, zoster<br>Invasion by head and neck tumors<br>Cerebellopontine angle tumor |
| VI. Abducens | Superior orbital fis-sure | Diplopia<br>Superior orbital fis-sure syndrome | Increased ICP<br>Brain stem lesion |
| VII. Facial | Stylomastoid foramen | Facial muscle weak-ness | Tumor metastasis along course of nerve<br>Cerebellopontine angle tumor<br>Idiopathic Bell's palsy<br>Zoster infection<br>Lyme disease<br>Infection of the temporal bone<br>Radiation injury is rare *continues* |

**Table 34-1** Cranial Nerves, Skull Foramina, Function, and Pathology *continued*

| Cranial Nerve | Skull Foramina or Fissure (Other Structures Present) | Symptoms | Differential Diagnosis |
|---|---|---|---|
| VIII. Auditory | Internal auditory canal | Loss of hearing<br>Loss of balance<br>Vertigo<br>Tinnitus | Cisplatin<br>Aminoglycosides<br>Leptomeningeal disease<br>Cerebellopontine angle tumor<br>Temporal bone metastasis |
| IX. Glosso-pharyngeal | Jugular foramen-pars nervosa (inferior petrosal sinuses) | Dysphagia<br>Loss of taste on posterior third of tongue<br>Hypotension and syncope (carotid body) | Direct extension of head and neck tumors |
| X. Vagus | Jugular foramen-pars vascularis (internal jugular vein, CN XI, arterial branches) | Dysphagia<br>Decreased gag reflex | Direct extension of head and neck tumors |
| XI. Spinal accessory | Jugular foramen<br>Foramen magnum-spinal segment (vertebral arteries and veins, anterior and posterior spinal arteries) | Trapezius weakness<br>Sternocleido-mastoid weakness<br>Vocal cord paralysis | |
| XII. Hypoglossal | Hypoglossal canal | Tongue weakness | Occipital condyle syndrome: unilateral pain, CN XII weakness, usually due to metastatic tumor |

ICP, intracranial pressure.

## Other Drugs

Aminoglycosides and loop diuretics can cause CN VIII injury with hearing loss, vertigo, and tinnitus.

## Radiation

Cranial neuropathies due to radiotherapy are less common than other CNS side effects of radiotherapy. Most CN injuries occur several months to years following radiotherapy, except injury to CN I and VIII, which is acute and common. Radiation damage to the cranial nerves generally is painless. Pain suggests tumor infiltration.

- CN I: alteration of smell.
- CN II: visual loss due to retinopathy, glaucoma, cataract, or optic neuropathy. Optic neuropathy presents as painless unilateral or bilateral visual loss occurring 7–26 months following exposure.
- CN III, IV, V, VI, VII injury rarely occurs.
- CN VIII: hearing loss or a sense of fullness in the ears during and after radiotherapy. This usually is due to serous otitis media as opposed to a true CN injury.
- Lower CN injury usually occurs following radiotherapy for head and neck tumors and is associated with fibrosis of surrounding structures.

## Infections

- Reactivation of varicella zoster virus infection ("shingles") can involve CN V and presents with dysesthetic pain and vesicular rash in the distribution of one or more branches of CN V. Rash is occasionally absent or subtle. Involvement of $V_1$ can cause visual loss due to corneal ulceration.
- Chronic meningitis can cause cranial neuropathies and should be considered when more than one CN is affected. VII is the most common CN affected. Etiologies include cryptococcus, tuberculosis, and other fungal infections.

## Direct Tumor Invasion or Compression

- Primary skull base tumors can directly invade and compress the cranial nerves. These include meningioma, nasopharyngeal carcinoma, and less commonly lymphoma, multiple myeloma, chondroma, sarcoma, and osteoma.
- Leptomeningeal metastasis should be considered especially when more than one CN is involved.

- Hematogenous metastases to the skull base usually are from lung, prostate, or breast primary tumors.
- Nerve sheath tumors (Schwannoma or neurofibroma) can affect any CN, especially VIII but also V (in Meckel's cave), IX, X, or XI.
- Nontumor causes of cranial neuropathies include fibrous dysplasia, sarcoidosis, Paget's disease, and histiocytosis X; they may be confused with neoplasms.

### Paraneoplastic

True cranial neuropathies do not occur due to paraneoplastic syndromes but cranial nerve symptoms can occur as a result of paraneoplastic myasthenia gravis, cerebellar degeneration, and the opsoclonus-myoclonus syndrome. Paraneoplastic vasculitic neuropathies can sometimes affect the CN.

## Syndromes Affecting More Than One Cranial Nerve

### Superior Orbital Fissure

- Affected structures within the superior orbital fissure include CN III, IV, $V_1$, VI, and the superior ophthalmic vein.
- Symptoms include headache (supra- or retro-orbital), diplopia due to oculomotor palsy, $V_1$ numbness, and exophthalmos.
- Tumors at this location usually are meningiomas, metastases, or carcinomas of the nasopharynx.

### Cavernous Sinus

- Structures within the cavernous sinus include CN III, IV, $V_1$ and $V_2$ (but not $V_3$), and VI.
- Symptoms include diplopia, exophthalmos, chemosis (erythema and swelling of the conjunctiva), and retro-orbital pain. Visual loss is possible.
- Typical tumors at this location are metastases or meningiomas.
- The differential diagnosis includes cavernous sinus thrombosis (due to infection or hypercoagulable states) and carotid-cavernous sinus-fistula.

### Cerebellopontine Angle

- Affected structures include CN V, VII, VIII, and sometimes IX and XII.
- Symptoms include hearing loss, vertigo, nystagmus, cerebellar symptoms, and brain stem symptoms.
- The differential diagnosis includes acoustic neuroma, meningioma, cholesteatoma, and metastases.

## *Jugular Foramen*

- Affected structures include CN IX, X, XI.
- Symptoms include hoarseness, dysphagia, posterior pharyngeal pain, and CN XI weakness.
- Glomus jugular tumor, neurinomas, chondromas, cholesteatoma, meningioma, and nasopharyngeal carcinoma occur in this region.

## *Apex of the Temporal Bone*

- Affected structures include CN V and VI.
- Symptoms include facial neuralgia and diplopia.
- Differential diagnosis includes inflammation, infection, or tumor.

## Suggested Reading

Adams RD, Victor M, Ropper AH. *Principles of Neurology* (6th ed). New York: McGraw-Hill, 1997.

Posner JB. *Neurologic Complications of Cancer.* Philadelphia: F.A. Davis, 1995.

# 35

# Deep Venous Thrombosis and Pulmonary Embolus

Thromboembolic complications (TEC) are an important cause of morbidity and mortality in patients with primary brain tumors and other cancers. Diagnosis depends on keeping a high index of suspicion. Despite concerns about intracranial hemorrhage, most patients with primary and metastatic brain tumors who develop TEC can be safely and successfully managed with heparin and warfarin. Thrombolytic agents are contraindicated. Inferior vena cava filters are used in conjunction with anticoagulation or in place of anticoagulation in certain circumstances. The new low-molecular-weight heparins can be used for acute therapy and may be appropriate for chronic therapy in some patients.

## Background and Prevention

- Deep venous thrombosis (DVT) has been reported in 27–72% of patients with primary brain tumors.
- This hypercoagulable state is thought to result from tumor/host interactions that alter hemostasis.
- Other potential risk factors for TEC in brain tumor patients include neurosurgery, chemotherapy exposure, immobility, age, congestive heart failure, obesity, progesterone or estrogen use, and prior thromboembolic disease.
- Patients are at particularly increased risk during perioperative periods, admissions for treatment, and other times of decreased mobility.
- During hospitalization, conservative measures, such as the use of compressive stockings or external compression boots, are warranted.

- Prophylaxis with subcutaneous heparin (5000 units bid) or one of the low-molecular-weight heparins should be considered standard therapy for hospitalized patients unless there is a contraindication.

## Presentation

- Symptoms and signs of TEC can be minor, absent, or atypical in presentation.
- Many patients with DVT are asymptomatic and then present with pulmonary embolus.
- There is a high incidence of concomitant, often asymptomatic, pulmonary embolus in brain tumor patients diagnosed with DVT.

## Diagnosis of Deep Venous Thrombosis

- Most (83%) DVTs in brain tumor patients occur in the femoral and popliteal veins. Less common sites include deep pelvic veins, upper extremities, and along indwelling catheters.
- Common symptoms include calf swelling, local pain, pain with ambulation, and calf cramps.
- Common signs include increased calf diameter, warmth, redness, edema, cord, distended superficial venous collaterals.
- Some patients have no clinical signs of DVT.

### Differential Diagnosis

The differential diagnosis for a swollen or painful leg includes edema, muscle pain due to rupture or strain, cramps or spasms due to upper motor neuron irritability or muscle weakness, cellulitis, radiculopathy, and lymphedema.

### Diagnostic Procedures

- Ultrasound (doppler)
  - Usually, ultrasound is the first diagnostic test. It is sensitive, rapidly available, and noninvasive.
  - False negative results occur if extensive collaterals have developed or there is a high degree of stenosis.
  - Ultrasound is more accurate for above the knee DVT than below the knee DVT.
- Venography
  - This technique is highly specific and may be needed if ultrasound studies are unrevealing or if the patient has had multiple prior DVTs.

- Risks include pain, inability to find a vein, infection, inflammatory reaction, and thrombogenesis.
- I 125-fibrinogen scan
  - This technique has been used extensively for research purposes and is highly sensitive.
  - Not useful for clinical decision making because the delay in accumulating sufficient isotope does not allow a timely diagnosis.

## Diagnosis of Pulmonary Embolus

- Pulmonary embolus (PE) always should be considered when a cancer patient presents with pulmonary symptoms, chest, or posterior thoracic pain.
- Pain syndromes may be atypical, and the "classic" pleuritic symptoms may be absent.
- Roughly 80–90% of PEs originate in the deep veins of the legs.
- Common symptoms include dyspnea (acute or subacute), thoracic pain (pleuritic or not), hemoptysis, and "back" pain.
- Signs may include atelectatic rales, local wheezes, pleural rub (if pleural effusion), fever, hypoxia, hypotension, or tachycardia.

### Diagnostic Procedures

- Chest X ray: wedge-shaped defect, nonspecific findings but usually normal.
- Electrocardiogram: normal or signs of pulmonary hypertension.
- Ventilation-perfusion scan (V/Q scan):
  - Normal perfusion scan nearly excludes PE.
  - Large mismatched defects: 90% probability of PE.
- Spiral computed tomography (CT) scan:
  - Study of choice when available.
  - Does not require patient cooperation with ventilation study.
  - Better differentiates PE from other pulmonary processes.

## Treatment

      The goals of treatment include preventing further propagation of clot, preventing pulmonary embolus, minimizing chronic venous insufficiency and postphlebitic syndromes, and preventing pulmonary hypertension. Contraindications to anticoagulant therapy are listed in Table 35-1.

**Table 35-1**  Contraindications to Anticoagulation of Cancer Patients

Bleeding diathesis

Active bleeding

Frequent severe falls

Major surgery or craniotomy within 30 days

Uncontrolled thrombocytopenia

Uncontrolled generalized seizures

## Anticoagulation

- Heparin (standard unfractionated heparin):
    - Binds to antithrombin III and inactivates several coagulation enzymes (thrombin, activated X, XII, XI, and IX). The serum t½ is 90–120 min and elimination generally is unaffected by renal or hepatic disease.
    - Dosage is through continuous IV infusion.
    - Goal is to maintain APPT of 1.5–2.0 times the control value. Table 35-2 provides a standard dosing nomogram for heparin use.
    - Starting dose: bolus 5000 units, then 1000 units/hour.
    - Heparin should be therapeutic for 24–48 hours prior to initiation of warfarin, then continued until patient is therapeutic on warfarin.
    - Significant risks include
      Clinically recognizable *bleeding* (5–8% of patients), generally from gastrointestinal or genitourinary sources.

**Table 35-2**  Raschke Weight-Based Heparin Dosing Guidelines

| APTT Ratio | Add Bolus Dose | Stop Infusion (minutes) | Infusion Rate Change (mL/hour)* | Rate Change (units/24 hours) |
|---|---|---|---|---|
| <1.5 | 500 | 0 | +3 | 3600 |
| 1.5–1.79 | 0 | 0 | +2 | 2400 |
| 1.8–2.5 | 0 | 0 | 0 | 0 |
| 2.51–3.1 | 0 | 0 | −1 | −1200 |
| 3.2–4.2 | 0 | 30 | −2 | −2400 |
| >4.2 | 0 | 60 | −3 | −3600 |

APTT, activated partial thromboplastin time.

*Starting dose = 5000 units heparin bolus and 1000 units/hour initial infusion; 1 ml/hour = 50 units/hour.

*Thrombocytopenia* normalizes after 3–5 days off heparin, and associated bleeding risk is <10%. Thrombosis can occur with heparin-induced thrombocytopenia. Other causes of thrombocytopenia should be considered, such as chemotherapy, sepsis, disseminated intravascular coagulation, immune-mediated thrombocytopenia, or bone marrow invasion by a tumor.

No increase in the rate of intracranial hemorrhage has been observed in brain tumor patients treated with anticoagulation vs. historical controls. The rate of spontaneous hemorrhage in both groups is roughly 2%.

- Warfarin:
  - After acute anticoagulation with heparin, patients are placed on warfarin.
  - Warfarin antagonizes vitamin K–dependent clotting proteins (prothrombin, protein C, protein S, and factors VII, IX, and X).
  - Warfarin is highly bound to plasma proteins and metabolized via the cytochrome P 450 system. There are *multiple drug interactions.*
  - Most patients require 4–5 days to become therapeutic on warfarin.
  - A starting dose of 5.0 mg PO per day is used with the goal of achieving an INR (international normalized ratio) of 2.0–3.0.
  - Risks: The risk of bleeding is related to the level of anticoagulation. When the INR is ≤2.0 the incidence is 4%; for INR 2.5–4.5, the incidence is 22%. The risk of bleeding also is greatest during the first month of treatment. Factors that increase bleeding risk include cerebrovascular disease, serious heart disease, liver dysfunction, renal insufficiency, concurrent aspirin and nonsteroidal anti-inflammatory drug (NSAID) use, but not age.
  - When corticosteroids and anticonvulsant agents are used in conjunction with warfarin, the drug interactions often are unpredictable. Close monitoring of the INR and anticonvulsant levels is needed.
- Low-molecular-weight heparins (LMWH):
  - LMWH has replaced standard heparin use for the prophylaxis and treatment of DVT in some patients.
  - Advantages compared with standard heparin include
  Better bioavailability, which allows fixed dosing.
  Subcutaneous dosing achieves therapeutic levels.
  Monitoring blood tests are not needed.
  Efficacy may be better than standard heparin in very high-risk patients.
  Lower incidence of osteoporosis.
  Lower incidence of heparin-induced thrombocytopenia.
  - Drawbacks of LMWH include
  Immediate reversal of anticoagulation using protamine sulfate is only 50–60% effective.

LMWH accumulates in patients with renal failure, requiring dose adjustment and monitoring of anti-Xa levels.

Cost.

– Indications for LMWH in neuro-oncology include

Prophylaxis of DVT: Enoxaparin 40 mg SC qd for patients with very high risk of DVT in the perioperative period.

Outpatient treatment of acute DVT: Enoxaparin 1 mg/kg SC q 12 hours for patients with documented acute DVT, patients who require interruption of warfarin treatment for procedures, and patients who develop new DVT while on therapeutic standard heparin or warfarin.

– Reversal of enoxaparin with protamine sulfate (PS): give 1 mg of PS per mg of enoxaparin. Additional doses may be needed, and PS can cause hypotension and anaphylaxis.

– Lumbar puncture and other invasive procedures should be avoided for 10 hours following the last dose of enoxaparin. The next dose should be delayed until 2 hours after the procedure.

### Inferior Vena Cava Filters

• Use of an inferior vena cava filter (IVCF) should be considered when
  – There are absolute contraindications to anticoagulation.
  – Anticoagulant therapy has failed.
  – The patient is expected to undergo future procedures or just had a procedure that makes anticoagulation contraindicated.
• Even with an IVCF in place, there is a significant risk of recurrent TEC so the use of low-dose anticoagulants (goal is an INR of 1.5–2.0) should be considered as an adjunct therapy.
• IVCF placement does not prevent pulmonary embolus (PE) from sites in the great thoracic vessels and upper extremities including clots that occur along indwelling catheters.
• Clots can develop on the proximal side of an IVCF and cause PE.
• Risks of an IVCF include persistent limb edema or pain, recurrent DVT or thrombophlebitis, and infection of the device.
• In general, patients treated with an IVCF without anticoagulation suffer a decreased quality of life compared with those who are treated with anticoagulation. Because most patients with an IVCF end up taking anticoagulants regardless, it is best to avoid IVCF placement if possible.

### Thrombolytic Agents

Due to an unacceptable rate of intracranial hemorrhage, the use of thrombolytic agents is absolutely contraindicated in patients with primary or metastatic brain tumors. This includes the streptokinase, urokinase, tissue plasminogen activator, and acylated lys-plasminogen-streptokinase activator complex.

## Thrombectomy

- Thrombectomy rarely is required and is reserved for threatened gangrene of the involved limb or saddle embolism of the main pulmonary artery with acute circulatory collapse that cannot be managed with aggressive supportive measures.
- Aggressive surgical intervention must be considered within the context of the patient's overall status.

## Duration of Treatment

Unless complications arise, patients should be anticoagulated for at least 3 months for DVT, 6 months for PE, and indefinitely if there are ongoing risk factors or recurrent TEC. Some physicians consider the presence of tumor an ongoing risk factor and favor chronic anticoagulation. IVCFs should be left in place unless complications require their removal.

## Suggested Reading

Constantini S, Kornowski R, Pomeranz S, Rappaport ZH. Thromboembolic phenomena in neurosurgical patients operated upon for primary and metastatic brain tumors. *Acta-Neurochir-Wien.* 1991;109(3–4):93–97.

Horton JD, Bushwick BM. Warfarin therapy: Evolving strategies in anticoagulation. *Am Fam Physician.* 1999;59(3):635–646.

Muchmore JH, Dunlap JN, Culicchia F, Kerstein MD. Deep vein thrombophlebitis and pulmonary embolism in patients with malignant gliomas. *South Med J.* 1989;82(11):1352–1356.

Mungall D, Anbe D, Forrester PL, et al. A prospective randomized comparison of the accuracy of computer-assisted versus GUSTO nomogram-directed heparin therapy. *Clin Pharmacol Ther.* 1994;55:591–596.

Raschke RA, Reilly BM, Guidry JR, et al. The weight-based heparin dosing nomongram compared with a "standard care" nomogram. A randomized controlled trial. *Ann Intern Med.* 1993;119:874–881.

# 36

# Depression and Anxiety

There is a high risk of major depression and anxiety disorders in cancer patients. Up to 25% of cancer patients meet diagnostic criteria for major depression, and many cancer patients exhibit some degree of anxiety. While there are no specific data regarding the prevalence of depression in brain tumor patients, it probably is similar. Making the diagnosis of depression in a cancer patient is challenging because of the overlap of symptoms of depression with signs and symptoms from the cancer and its treatments. Patients with primary and metastatic brain tumors are particularly challenging because many have affective symptoms due to their tumors. Depression is a significant complication of cancer because it decreases the quality of life and depressed patients are less likely to pursue active treatment. Diagnosing and treating depression in cancer patients can enhance their quality of life and may even improve survival by promoting cooperation with therapy, improving immune function, and improving the patient's nutritional status.

## Depression vs. Anxiety

*Depression* is a state characterized by depressed mood, anhedonia, loss of interest, and worthlessness. Patients with severe depression may be occupied by thoughts of death and have vegetative symptoms such as insomnia and anorexia.

*Anxiety* is a general state of apprehension and dread with no identifiable source. Anxiety is distinguished from *fear*, which has a specific source (e.g., fear of pain). Anxiety may occur as a component of several affective disorders, particularly depression.

## Risk Factors for Depression in Cancer Patients

- Advanced stage of cancer or poor prognosis.
- Relapse after a period of remission.
- Pre-existing mood disorder.
- History of alcoholism.
- Use of medications with depressive side effects (Table 36-1).
- Uncontrolled pain.
- Poor performance status.
- Loss of mobility or independence.
- Disfigurement.
- Exhaustion and fatigue.
- Social isolation.

## Diagnosing Depression in Cancer Patients

*Somatic symptoms* such as anorexia, fatigue, insomnia, weight loss, and decreased libido are important for diagnosing depression in healthy patients. These symptoms are less specific when considering depression in cancer patients, since they are common symptoms of cancer and cancer therapies.

*Affective symptoms*, such as lack of initiative and inattentiveness, commonly associated with depression also are common symptoms of primary and metastatic brain tumors. Other symptoms such as withdrawal and sadness are part of an appropriate response to the diagnosis of cancer; however, when severe or unremitting they may indicate depression.

*Distinguishing symptoms* helpful in diagnosing depression in cancer patients include

- Feelings of worthlessness.
- Guilt.
- Feelings of being a burden.
- Suicidal ideation.
- Prolonged crying.

The diagnosis of depression may be delayed or missed because of clinician, caregiver, or patient biases.

*Clinicians* may

- Wrongfully attribute depressive symptoms to medications.
- Be reluctant to ask about depressive symptoms because they are busy and lack expertise in managing depression.
- Be concerned about upsetting the patient.
- Feel that depression is normal in a cancer patient.

**Table 36-1**  Drugs with Side Effects of Depression or Anxiety

| Drug Class | Specific Agents |
|---|---|
| Chemotherapeutic agents | Procarbazine<br>Vinca alkaloids (uncommon)<br>L-asparaginase<br>Tamoxifen (uncommon)<br>Interferons |
| Anticonvulsant agents | Phenobarbital (depression or agitation)<br>Valproic acid[a]<br>Carbamazepine[a]<br>Phenytoin<br>Benzodiazepines |
| Cardiac | Beta-blockers<br>Clonidine<br>Digitalis<br>Diltiazem<br>Nifedipine<br>Reserpine |
| Analgesics | Opiates |
| Antiemetics and gastrointestinal medications | Benzodiazepines<br>Metoclopromide<br>H-2 blockers, ranitidine, cimetidine |
| Amphetamine | Abuse or withdrawal |
| Pulmonary medications | Theophylline (anxiety)<br>Albuterol (anxiety) |
| Sedatives and tranquilizers | Lorazepam[b]<br>Diazepam[b]<br>Triazolam[b]<br>Alprazolam[b] |
| Neuroleptic drugs | Haloperidol |
| Others | Caffeine<br>Corticosteroids<br>Baclofen<br>Bromocriptine<br>L-dopa |

[a]More often, valproic acid and carbamezapine stabilize mood.

[b]The benzodiazepines can cause depression and sedation; however, some patients develop paradoxical agitation and anxiety.

- Expect the patient to bring up the issue of depression without being asked.
- Feel sad while talking to the patient about depression.

*Patients* may

- Not want to further burden their caregivers.
- Feel helpless and hopeless.
- Not want to be labeled a "psychiatric" patient.
- Feel that depression is a normal reaction.
- Be embarrassed to admit to depression with family members or friends present.

## Approaches to Management of Depression and Anxiety

### Consider Contributing Medical Conditions and Medications

- Table 36-1 lists some commonly used medications that can cause or contribute to depression and anxiety.
- Medical conditions that may cause or contribute to depression include hyponatremia, anemia, hypo- or hypercalcemia, hypothyroidism, adrenal insufficiency, poor nutrition, and chronic infection.
- Medical conditions that may cause or contribute to anxiety include respiratory distress, hypoxia, pulmonary embolism, uncontrolled pain, impending sepsis, hypoglycemia, hypocalcemia.

### Laboratory Investigations

Check patient's levels of

- Electrolytes.
- Glucose.
- Calcium.
- Complete blood count with red blood cell indexes.
- Thyroid function tests.
- Oxygen saturation (for anxiety).

### Pharmacologic Treatment

Medications useful for treating depression and anxiety are summarized in Table 36-2.

- Appropriate treatment of pain and other disturbing symptoms is critical in the management of depression and anxiety.

**Table 36-2**  Pharmacologic Treatments for Depression and Anxiety
in Cancer Patients

| Class of Drug | Drug and Dosing | Comments |
|---|---|---|
| Tricyclic antidepressant agents | Amitryptiline: Starting dose, 10–25 mg Increase by 10–25 mg increments every 3–4 days, up to 125–150 mg Nortriptiline (similar dosing) | Helpful for insomnia May help pain control May cause urinary retention and constipation Causes dry mouth |
| Stimulants | Methylphenidate: 10 mg in A.M. and 5 mg at noon | Rapid onset May cause anorexia Counteracts sedation from opiates |
| Benzodiazepines | Lorazepam | Useful when anxiety present Some anticonvulsant effect |

- For depression, stimulants can be particularly helpful because of their rapid onset of action and lack of sedating effects.
- Associated insomnia often requires specific treatment in addition to antidepressant agents. Approaches to insomnia are covered in Chapter 44.
- Anxiety often requires specific treatment. Benzodiazepines usually are helpful and have the added benefits of treating nausea and raising the seizure threshold. Stimulant agents should be avoided.
- Occasional patients have paradoxical agitation with benzodiazepines.
- Monoamine oxidase inhibitors are rarely used for depression anymore, and they must be avoided in patients using Procarbazine.
- Tricyclic antidepressant agents may lower the seizure threshold. Wellbutrin commonly lowers the seizure threshold and should be avoided if intracranial pathology is present. The new selective serotonin reuptake inhibitors do not alter seizure threshold; neither does Doxepin.

## Counseling

- The treating physician should ensure that the patient has a realistic understanding of the tumor, its treatment, and prognosis.
- Some patients equate the diagnosis of cancer with a terminal condition and may develop a more positive outlook if given accurate information about their chances of survival.

- For some patients, contact with patients having a similar diagnosis is helpful.
- Support groups allow patients to discuss their problems in coping with cancer with others.
- Foster patient's coping skills, self-reliance, and self-esteem.
- Enlist support of family and friends.
- Psychotherapy from a psychiatrist or psychologist may be needed.

## Suggested Reading

Bottomley A. Psychosocial problems in cancer care: A brief review of common problems. *J Psychiatr Ment Health Nurs.* 1997;4(5):323–331.

Holland J (ed). *Psych-Oncology.* New York: Oxford University Press, 1998.

Kuzel R. Management of depression: Current trends in primary care. *Postgrad Med.* 1996;99(5):179–192.

Massie MJ, Gagnon P, Holland JC. Depression and suicide in patients with cancer. *J Pain Symptom Manage.* 1994;9(5):325–340.

McCoy DM. Treatment considerations for depression in patients with significant medical comorbidity. *J Fam Pract.* 1996;43(6 suppl):S35–S44.

McDaniel JS, Musselman DL, Porter MR, et al. Depression in patients with cancer: Diagnosis, biology, and treatment. *Arch Gen Psychiatry.* 1995;52(2): 89–99.

Olin J, Masand P. Psychostimulants for depression in hospitalized cancer patients. *Psychosomatics.* 1996;37(1):57–62.

Schulberg HC, Katon WJ, Simon GE, Rush AJ. Best clinical practice: Guidelines for managing major depression in primary medical care. *J Clin Psychiatry.* 1999;60(suppl 7):19–26.

Spiegel D. Cancer and depression. *Brit J of Psychiatry-Supplement.* 1996;30: 109–116.

Valente SM, Saunders JM. Diagnosis and treatment of major depression among people with cancer. *Cancer Nurs.* 1997;20(3):168–177.

Visser MR, Smets EM. Fatigue, depression and quality of life in cancer patients: How are they related? *Support Care Cancer.* 1998;6(2):101–108.

# 37

# Differential Diagnosis of Brain Tumor Progression

Tumor progression frequently is assumed to be the cause of declining functional status in brain tumor patients. Other conditions, both neurologic and nonneurologic, may cause such a decline and should be considered as contributing factors, particularly when imaging studies fail to demonstrate tumor progression. A list of diagnostic considerations is provided. Most of these conditions are covered in more detail elsewhere in this book.

## Neurologic Conditions

- Anticonvulsant toxicity.
- Cisplatin neuropathy.
- Vincristine neuropathy.
- Central nervous system (CNS) infection.
- Parkinsonism, idiopathic or drug related.
- Procarbazine encephalopathy.
- Radiation encephalopathy or necrosis.
- Steroid myopathy.
- Subclinical seizures.
- Subdural hematoma.
- Other unrelated neurologic conditions.

## Nonneurologic Conditions

- Adrenal insufficiency.
- Congestive heart failure.

- Depression.
- Fatigue from chemotherapy, anemia, or radiotherapy.
- Hypercarbia.
- Hypothyroidism.
- Hypoxia.
- Pulmonary embolism.
- Systemic infection.

# 38

# Fatigue and Weakness

Fatigue and weakness are common symptoms in cancer patients and contribute significantly to a lessened quality of life. The causes often are multifactorial, with some factors being treatable and some not. The goals of evaluation are to identify conditions amenable to treatment and conditions that may be important from a prognostic or management standpoint. Distinguishing between fatigue and true muscular weakness helps guide the evaluation. Patients may use a variety of words to report fatigue including weakness, exhaustion, tiredness, weariness, sleepiness, drowsiness, or loss of energy. Furthermore, patients may report fatigue when they actually suffer from weakness, somnolence, shortness of breath, or depression. Some patients many even use the terms numbness and weakness interchangeably. A careful history and physical examination helps determine precisely what the patient is experiencing and directs further evaluation.

## Definitions and Guidelines

*Fatigue* refers to a persistent feeling of poor energy and lessened capacity for activity.

- Fatigue may not improve with rest or may be present at rest.
- Fatigue interferes with desired activities and personal enjoyment.
- Although fatigued patients may require more sleep, fatigue should be distinguished from *somnolence*, which is a disorder of arousal (see Chapter 45).

*Weakness* refers to a loss of muscle power or strength and becomes apparent with attempted activity.

- Weakness with hyperactive reflexes suggests *epidural spinal cord compression* (see Chapter 5) or intracranial pathology.

- A pattern of *proximal muscle weakness* with preserved reflexes suggests a myopathy or myasthenia gravis.
  - Patients with proximal lower extremity weakness typically have trouble getting out of a low chair, off the toilet, or going up stairs.
  - Patients with proximal upper extremity weakness typically have trouble with activities requiring the arms to be held overhead such as putting away dishes or reaching for objects overhead.
- A pattern of *distal weakness* with hypoactive reflexes suggests a neuropathy.
  - Weakness due to neuropathy usually is associated with sensory symptoms.
  - Patients with distal lower extremity weakness typically have trouble standing on their heels, have difficulty walking up stairs, or may trip over their toes when walking.
  - Patients with distal upper extremity weakness typically have difficulty opening jars, buttoning clothing, or other activities requiring hand strength.
- Respiratory weakness can occur with a variety of neurologic conditions.

## Evaluation and Management

Table 38-1 summarizes some important causes of weakness in cancer patients along with guidelines for management.

## Examination

In particular, look for asterixis, hepatic failure, muscle wasting, anemia, and pallor.

## Laboratory Investigations

Check the levels of the following:

Complete blood count.
Electrolytes, calcium, magnesium.
Glucose.
Adrenal evaluation, as appropriate.
Thyroid-stimulating hormone.
Drug levels, as appropriate.

## Practical Management

- Address treatable causes (see Table 38-1).

**Table 38-1** Causes of Weakness in Cancer Patients

| Etiology | Site of Pathology | Clinical Considerations | Evaluation | Management |
|---|---|---|---|---|
| Cachectic myopathy | Muscle | Proximal > distal weakness, preserved reflexes | Exclude other diagnoses | Improve nutritional status and conditioning |
| Corticosteroid myopathy | Muscle | Proximal > distal weakness, preserved reflexes | Exclude other diagnoses | Improve conditioning, physical therapy |
| Disuse myopathy | Muscle | Proximal > distal weakness | History of bedrest or decline in activity level | Increase activity, physical therapy |
| Drug-induced myopathy | Muscle | Proximal > distal weakness, preserved reflexes | Review recent medications | Withdraw medication, if possible |
| Electrolyte imbalances | Muscle and peripheral nerve | K<br>Ca<br>Na<br>Mg | Serum K<br>Serum, ionized Ca<br>Serum Na<br>Serum Mg | Treat specific imbalance |
| Intracranial process | Brain:<br>Metastasis<br>Stroke<br>Infection | Lateralizing weakness, ± sensory symptoms, ± cognitive symptoms, upper motor neuron signs | CT or MRI of brain | Treat underlying process<br>Treat associated problems:<br>Increased ICP<br>Headaches<br>Spasticity |
| Lambert-Eaton syndrome | Neuromuscular junction (pre-synaptic) | Muscle weakness improves following use, small-cell lung cancer | NCV/EMG with repetitive stimulation | Treat underlying tumor |
| Mononeuropathies | Single peripheral nerve | Localized weakness in the distribution of a single nerve, may have associated sensory symptoms or pain (e.g., carpal tunnel syndrome) | Clinical exam, nerve conduction studies, and EMG | Specific for the syndrome |

*continues*

**Table 38-1**   Causes of Weakness in Cancer Patients   *continued*

| Etiology | Site of Pathology | Clinical Considerations | Evaluation | Management |
|---|---|---|---|---|
| Myasthenia gravis | Neuromuscular junction (postsynaptic) | Muscle weakness worsens with use and fatigue | EMG with repetitive stimulation | Corticosteroids, acetylcholinesterase inhibitors, plasmapheresis |
| Peripheral neuropathy | Peripheral nerves | Symmetrical motor and sensory deficits | Chapter 48 | |
| Plexopathy | Brachial or lumbar plexus | Sensory and motor deficits in a single limb | Chapter 48 | |
| Polymyalgia rheumatica | Muscle | Major complaint is muscle pain and stiffness, weakness is minimal | Elevated ESR | Corticosteroids Pain medications |
| Polymyositis and dermatomyositis | Muscle | Pain and weakness, rash with dermatomyositis | Consider EMG Consider muscle biopsy ESR | Corticosteroids and other immunosuppressants |
| Radiculopathy | Nerve root | Weakness in the distribution of a single nerve root | Chapter 48 | Chapter 48 |
| Spinal cord compression | Spinal cord | Back pain, weakness below the compression level, sphincter dysfunction | Chapter 5 | Chapter 5 |

EMG, electromyography; NCV, nerve conduction velocity; ICP, intracranial pressure; ESR, erythrocyte sedimentation rate; CT, computed tomography; MRI, magnetic resonance imaging.

- Help patient set priorities in activities, plan for rest, exercise (which helps some patients, especially if there is a strong psychosocial component), improve sleep quality.
- Conserve energy for activities that are important to him or her.

## Suggested Reading

Dropcho EJ, Soong S-J. Steroid-induced weakness in patients with primary brain tumors. *Neurology.* 1991;41:1235–1239.

Regnard CFB, Mannix KA. Weakness and fatigue in advanced cancer: A flow diagram. *Palliative Med.* 1992;6(2):253.

# 39

# Fever and Neutropenia

The dose-limiting toxicity for many patients receiving chemotherapy is neutropenia. These patients have an increased risk of serious or life-threatening infection that is dependent on the severity of the neutropenia. Those who develop fever in the face of neutropenia must be evaluated and treated promptly and decisively. Failure to do so may lead to unacceptable morbidity or mortality in someone who otherwise is responding well to treatment.

## Absolute Neutrophil Count

The absolute neutrophil count (ANC) may be calculated

$$ANC \text{ (cells/}\mu l) = \text{leukocyte count (cells/}\mu l) \times \% \text{ (neutrophils + bands)}$$

An absolute neutrophil count of $\leq 500/\mu l$ is associated with a dramatic increase in the rate of serious infection. A temperature of $\geq 38.5°C$ is a call for action. Although these numbers may serve as guidelines, there is no substitute for evaluating the ill patient who does not meet these arbitrary criteria.

## Preparation

One philosopher noted that, "Discovery comes to the prepared mind." When treatment with chemotherapy is started, the patient and family must be educated about the signs and symptoms of infection. Many patients will ignore minor symptoms, attributing them to a cold or other respiratory infection, when they have the earliest signs of a serious infection. The lines of communication must be clear, so that individuals know whom to contact. We encourage patients to call promptly; they must not wait until "office" hours for fear of bothering someone. Patients must be told specifically that the highest risk is *not* temporally related to the dose of chemotherapy but may be 1–2 weeks *after* the treatment (3–8 weeks after nitrosourea agents).

All patients should observe good personal hygiene, and caregivers should carefully wash their hands before contact with the patient. This simple intervention often is overlooked.

## Evaluation

When a chemotherapy patient develops fever, he or she must be seen promptly. Historical clues relating to a possible source of the fever should be sought, and a focused physical examination is necessary. The ANC should be determined. If a fever is documented and the ANC is ≤500/µl, blood cultures should be obtained. If a venous access device is present, cultures should also be obtained from this line. If urinary symptoms are present, appropriate cultures should be procured. Pulmonary symptoms mandate a chest radiograph.

## Treatment

After the initial evaluation is complete, antibiotics should be started *promptly.* The first dose should be given ASAP. If routine channels are used, it can be hours between the time an order is written and the actual antibiotic is ordered. Time can be of the essence if one is dealing with an organism such as *Pseudomonas aeruginosa.* If no clear-cut source for infection can be found, it is our policy to initiate therapy with a regimen able to control *P. aeruginosa.* Initial treatment could include

1. Ceftazadime 1 gram IV q 8 hours *or*
2. Imipenem 500 mg IV q 6 hours *or*
3. Piperacillin 3 grams IV q 4 hours *and* Gentamicin 1.7mg/kg IV q 8 hrs (loading dose = 2 mg/kg).

The actual drugs chosen probably are less important than the rapidity with which antibiotic treatment is begun. Cost, local infection patterns, hospital-specific sensitivity patterns, and nursing convenience may affect the initial choice. As either single agent, ceftazadime or imipenem, is associated with a good outcome and as they are relatively simple to administer, we usually start with a single-agent antipseudomonal agent unless clinical circumstances suggest another approach. When culture results and sensitivities are available, the antibiotic regimen can be tailored accordingly.

Although empiric therapy should include coverage for *P. aeruginosa,* the clinical situation may dictate other treatment as well. If a central line or IV site is red and swollen, coverage for *Staphylococcus aureus* should be included. An obvious oral or perirectal infection or intra-abdominal symptoms may require anaerobic coverage. In patients on steroids, evidence for a fungal infection such as thrush or *Candida esophagitis* requires antifungal therapy. *Pneumocystis carinii* pneumonia also occurs in patients on steroids and initially may cause only minimal symptoms.

Initial therapy typically is given intravenously while the patient is hospitalized. Recent randomized trials suggest that some highly compliant patients who meet predetermined criteria rendering them at low risk may be treated with empiric oral therapy using ciprofloxacin and amoxicillin-clavulanate.

### Growth Factors

Recombinant growth factors can accelerate the recovery of neutrophils from chemotherapy-induced nadirs and also can be used prophylactically after chemotherapy in patients who have previously had infections in the face of neutropenia. The American Society of Clinical Oncology (ASCO) has published practice guidelines for their use (see the Suggested Reading section). The two available growth factors are G-CSF (filgramastim) and GM-CSF (sargramostim). The G-CSF dose is 5 µg/kg/day, given either subcutaneously or intravenously. Nonreusable vial sizes of 300 or 480 µg are available, and the full vial should be given. The GM-CSF dose is 250 µg/kg/day. Myeloid growth factors should be considered in patients with febrile neutropenia and certain high-risk features: poor performance status, hypotension, pneumonia, or multiorgan dysfunction. To preserve dose-intensity, patients who have had an episode of fever in the face of neutropenia may be given G-CSF prophylactically with subsequent cycles of chemotherapy. This intervention will reduce the duration of associated neutropenia and decrease the risk of serious infection.

### Suggested Reading

ASCO Ad Hoc Colony-Stimulating Factor Guidelines Expert Panel. American Society of Clinical Oncology recommendations for the use of hematopoietic colony-stimulating factors: Evidence-based, clinical practice guidelines. *J Clin Oncol.* 1994;12:2471–2508.

Freifeld A, Marchigiani D, Walsh T, et al. A double-blind comparison of empirical oral and intravenous antibiotic therapy for low-risk febrile patients with neutropenia during cancer chemotherapy. *N Engl J Med.* 1999;341: 305–311.

Freifeld AG, Walsh T, Marshall D, et al. Monotherapy for fever and neutropenia in cancer patients: A randomized comparison of ceftazidime versus imipenem. *J Clin Oncol.* 1995;13:165–176.

Gilbert DN, Moellering RC Jr, Sande MA. *The Sanford Guide to Antimicrobial Therapy 2001* (31st ed). Hyde Park, VT: Antimicrobial Therapy, Inc., 2001.

Hughes WT, Armstrong D, Bodey GP, et al. Guidelines for the use of antimicrobial agents in neutropenic patients with unexplained fever. *J Infectious Dis.* 1990;161:381–396.

Kern WV, Cometta A, de Bock R, et al. Oral versus intravenous empirical antimicrobial therapy for fever in patients with granulocytopenia who are receiving cancer chemotherapy. *N Engl J Med.* 1999;341:312–318.

Ozer H, Miller LL, Schiffer CA, Winn RJ, Smith TJ. American Society of Clinical Oncology update of recommendations for the use of hematopoietic colony-stimulating factors: Evidence-based, clinical practice guidelines. *J Clin Oncol.* 1996;14:1957–1960.

Pizzo PA. Management of fever in patient with cancer and treatment-induced neutropenia. *N Engl J Med.* 1993;328:1323–1332.

Pizzo PA, Hathorn JW, Hiemenz J, et al. A randomized trial comparing ceftazadime alone with combination antibiotic therapy in patients with fever and neutropenia. *N Engl J Med.* 1986;315:552–558.

# 40

# Gait Disturbances

Gait disturbances are common causes of disability and loss of independence in patients with primary and metastatic brain tumors, spinal cord tumors, and systemic cancers. Etiologies include both neurologic and nonneurologic disorders. A localization-based approach to diagnosis is presented.

## Frontal Lobe Ataxia or Gait Apraxia

### Clinical Features

- Flexion posture, slightly wide base.
- Short shuffling steps.
- Turns accomplished with multiple small steps.
- Difficulty turning over in bed.
- No loss of sensation or muscle strength.
- Spasticity of legs on examination.
- No cerebellar signs on examination.
- Associated frontal lobe dementia and urinary urgency or incontinence.

### Etiologies and Evaluation

- Bilateral frontal lobe tumors (malignant glioma) or large unilateral tumors (glioma, meningioma, metastasis) that compress the contralateral frontal lobe.
- Multiple infarcts.
- Radiation injury.
- Pick's disease.

## Hydrocephalic Gait

### Clinical Features

- Wide base.
- Diminished cadence and height of steps.
- Short shuffling steps.
- Diminished arm swing.
- Other parkinsonian features are absent.

### Etiologies and Evaluation

- Obstructive hydrocephalus:
  - Headache, nausea or vomiting.
  - Ventricular dilation on computed tomography (CT) or magnetic resonance imaging (MRI) scan.
  - Tumor of cerebellum or ventricular pathways.
- Nonobstructing (communicating) hydrocephalus:
  - Headache, nausea and vomiting less common than with obstruction.
  - All ventricles are dilated on CT or MRI scan.
  - Consider chronic meningitis or leptomeningeal tumor.
- Normal pressure hydrocephalus:
  - Memory loss.
  - Urinary incontinence.
  - Ventricles may be significantly dilated on CT or MRI scans.

## Gait Problems Due to Lesions in the Cerebral Hemispheres

- *Bilateral white matter injury* can cause a spastic paraparesis, but other features are more prominent, such as dementia and hyperreflexia. The clinical picture is similar to hydrocephalus.
  - Radiation encephalopathy.
  - Methotrexate encephalopathy.
  - White matter infections: cytomegalovirus, progressive multifocal leukoencephalopathy.
  - Multiple metastases.
  - Multiple infarcts.
  - Multiple sclerosis.
  - Inherited leukoencephalopathy (rare).

- *Unilateral or bilateral parietal lobe lesions* can cause gait abnormalities due to neglect, which affects the contralateral side of the body. This is more evident with right hemispheric lesions. Patients may veer to the right or bump into objects on the left side and be unaware of their deficit.
- *Cortical visual loss* can cause gait abnormalities due to a hemianopsia. If there is parietal involvement the patient may be unaware of the deficit (neglect).

### Cerebellar Gait

#### Clinical Features

- Patient complains of loss of balance, unsteadiness, and falls.
- Gait is wide based with lateral instability and irregular steps.
- Patient has most difficulty when standing up from seated position, turning, and stopping.
- Patient has severe difficulty with tandem walking.
- If severe, the patient is unable to stand upright without support.
- Other signs of ataxia may be present such as appendicular ataxia, ataxia of voice, or tremor.

#### Etiologies and Evaluation

- Differential diagnosis includes cerebellar tumors, stroke, multiple sclerosis, and paraneoplastic cerebellar degeneration.
- Ataxia involving the legs and trunk but not the arms or speech suggests a lesion in the cerebellar vermis.
- Chemotherapy agents that may be the cause: high-dose IV cytarabine (acute, reversible), 5-fluorouracil.
- Medications that may be the cause: phenytoin, procarbazine, antihistamines, antidepressants.
- Infection: varicella.

### Festinating Gait

#### Clinical Features

- Festination is involuntary hastening of gait resulting in short steps and the feet barely clear the floor.
- Rigidity and shuffling.
- Center of gravity shifts forward and patient may fall forward.
- Parkinsonian features usually are present, including tremor, masked facies, decreased blinking, and flexion posture.

### Etiologies and Evaluation

- Idiopathic Parkinson's disease.
- Parkinsonism due to medications:
  - Metoclopromide.
  - Antipsychotic agents.
  - Valproic acid.
- Parkinsonism due to cerebral injury.

## Spastic Gait

### Clinical Features

- Legs are stiff with minimal flexion at ankle, knee, and hip.
- Leg swings laterally with forward movement, circumduction.
- Audible "scuffling" of foot on floor.
- Hemiparesis: The arm on the same side is also stiff and does not swing.
- Paraparesis: Both legs are stiff, resulting in a "scissors" gait.
- Increased reflexes and spasticity on examination.

### Etiologies and Evaluation

- Hemiparesis:
  - Unilateral cerebral lesion: tumor, stroke, or abscess.
  - Asymmetrical spinal cord lesion (uncommon).
- Paraparesis (see Chapter 5):
  - Myelopathy: spinal cord tumor, pernicious anemia, multiple sclerosis, infection, or paraneoplastic (anti-Hu).
  - Myelopathy due to intrathecal chemotherapy.
  - Radiation myelitis.
  - Epidural hematoma, following lumbar puncture.
  - Central disc herniation (not always painful).
  - Bilateral cerebral white matter injury: leukoencephalopathy, multiple sclerosis, anoxic injury, cerebral palsy, and hereditary conditions.

## Sensory Ataxia

### Clinical Features

- Wide base.
- Legs slap or stamp the floor and movements are jerky.
- Patient watches legs to guide movement; gait is worse without visual cues.

- Romberg's sign is present: When the patient is asked to stand with feet together and eyes closed, marked swaying and even falling is observed.
- Loss of position sense.
- Decreased or absent leg reflexes.

## Etiologies and Evaluation

- Abnormality of joint position sense due to lesion of afferent nerves, posterior roots, posterior columns of spinal cord, or bilateral parietal lobes (rare).
- Due to chemotherapy agents.
  - Common: cisplatin, vincristine, and taxol.
  - Less common: procarbazine, suramin, and cytarabine.
- Paraneoplastic sensory neuronopathy (anti-Hu syndrome).
- Spinal cord compression (of posterior columns).
- Sensory polyneuropathy (see Chapter 48).
- Multiple sclerosis.
- Tabes dorsalis (central nervous system syphilis).
- Hereditary spinocerebellar degeneration.
- Subacute combined degeneration (vitamin $B_{12}$ deficiency).

## Steppage Gait Due to Distal Motor Weakness

### Clinical Features

- Weakness of dorsiflexion and eversion at ankle.
- Foot drop.
- Exaggerated flexion at the hip needed to clear the foot off the ground with forward swing.
- Slapping sound as foot strikes the floor.
- Normal to diminished reflexes depending on the etiology.

## Etiologies and Evaluation

- Compression of common peroneal nerve at head of fibula: associated with sensory loss on the dorsum of foot, reflexes are normal.
- Polyneuropathy: associated with stocking-glove distribution sensory loss and hypoactive reflexes.
- Motor neuropathies often are hereditary. In cancer patients, they may be due to vincristine.
- L5 radiculopathy: degenerative spine disease, metastasis with compression of L5 nerve root, leptomeningeal metastasis.

## Waddling Gait

### Clinical Features

- Waddling of gait due to hip girdle weakness.
- Difficulty rising from low chair or toilet.

### Etiologies and Evaluation (see Chapter 38)

- Relates to proximal muscle weakness, which may also involve the upper extremities.
- Steroid myopathy.
- Muscular dystrophy.
- Other myopathies.

## Gait Deterioration with Exertion

- Increasing weakness with exertion or persistent use is common in cancer patients due to generalized fatigue and deconditioning.
- Myasthenia gravis, a neuromuscular junction defect, can be a paraneoplastic syndrome (malignant thymoma).
- Claudication due to vascular disease results in severe leg pain and calf cramping with ambulation. Patients improve with rest and motor strength and control are normal at rest.
- Spinal stenosis ("pseudoclaudication") can cause exertional back and leg pain that is relieved by stopping and bending forward at the waist.

## Hysterical

- Legs are advanced in a jerky and grossly ataxic fashion.
- Leg may be dragged on the floor or pushed ahead of the patient.
- Extreme dystonic postures.
- Wild lurching.
- Hysterical patients may manifest significant abnormalities of gait but then use appropriate postural mechanisms to right themselves and rarely fall.

## Antalgic (Painful) Gait

### Clinical Features

- Pain in the feet, legs, hips, or spine can cause gait difficulties due to increased pain with weight-bearing and limb movement.
- Painful neuropathy.

- Bone metastases.
- Fractures due to osteoporosis (accelerated by steroids).
- Arthritis.
- Soft tissue pain.
- Epidural spine metastasis.

## Suggested Reading

Adams RD, Victor M, Ropper AH. *Principles of Neurology* (6th ed). New York: McGraw-Hill, 1997.

# 41

# Headaches

Headaches occur in about half the patients with primary and metastatic brain tumors and account for a reduction in quality of life if not managed appropriately. The "classic" symptoms associated with brain tumor headaches are experienced primarily by patients with increased intracranial pressure. Such patients experience positional headaches that are moderate to severe in intensity and associated with vomiting or other symptoms of raised intracranial pressure. More commonly, patients with brain tumors experience less severe headaches of a nonspecific nature. New headaches should be carefully evaluated in patients with known malignancies, as they may be the initial manifestation of serious intracranial pathology. Headaches due to other factors should be carefully excluded.

## Etiology and Risk Factors

- Headaches are thought to arise from traction, pressure, ischemia, or invasion of extracranial and intracranial pain-sensitive structures.
- Extracranial pain-sensitive structures include
  - The arteries at the base of the head and neck.
  - Periosteum of the skull.
  - Scalp and galea.
  - Muscles of the scalp, face, and neck and their associated fascias.
  - Mucosal surfaces.
- Intracranial pain-sensitive structures include
  - The large arteries at the base of the brain and dura mater (carotid, vertebral, and basilar).
  - Venous sinuses.
  - Dura located near the venous sinuses and large vessels.
  - Upper cervical nerves (C2 and C3).
  - Cranial nerves V, IX, X, and XI.

- Structures known not to be pain sensitive include
  - Brain parenchyma.
  - Ependyma.
  - Choroid plexus.
  - Intracranial periosteum.
  - Extracranial veins.
  - Arachnoid granulations.

## Contributing Factors

Factors that tend to increase the likelihood of headaches in brain tumor patients include

- Larger tumor size.
- Faster growing tumors.
- Obstruction of cerebrospinal fluid (CSF) pathways.
- Prior history of headaches.

## Clinical Evaluation

### History

The most important step in evaluating the headache patient is obtaining a history. The diagnosis of headache type guides therapy. Important factors to ascertain include these:

- Location of headache.
- Frequency and duration of headache.
- Type of pain (dull ache, throbbing, burning, tingling).
- Associated symptoms (nausea, vomiting, tinnitus, photophobia).
- Diurnal variation (morning headaches, headache during sleep).
- Precipitating factors (stress, position changes, Valsalva maneuver).
- Alleviating factors (rest or sleep, dark, medications, lying down, standing up, vomiting).
- Warning symptoms or aura.
- Family history of headaches (85% of migraine patients have a positive family history).
- Medications and medical history.

### Physical and Neurologic Examination

The general physical examination may disclose signs related to the etiology of the headaches. Specific attention should be paid to the blood pressure, fundoscopic exam (for papilledema), meningeal signs, scalp, neck, or temporal artery tenderness. The neurologic exam may be helpful in localizing a possible intracranial lesion, but a normal exam does not exclude serious intracranial pathology.

### "Brain tumor headaches"

- "Classic" brain tumor headaches are
  - Holocranial.
  - Throbbing or nonthrobbing.
  - Positional (increased supine, bending over).
  - Nocturnal or early morning.
  - Constant and progressive.
  - Moderate to severe in intensity.
  - Associated with vomiting.
  - Increased intensity with cough, sneeze, or other Valsalva maneuvers.
  - Associated with overt or subtle symptoms of increased intracranial pressure (ICP).
- These features occur in a minority (17%) of patients with primary and metastatic brain tumors and generally are associated with raised intracranial pressure. Treatment is directed at decreasing intracranial pressure (see Chapter 43), and narcotics may be needed to control pain. When these headaches are progressive and associated with other ominous signs and symptoms of increased intracranial pressure, management will include hospital admission and aggressive treatment.

### Nonspecific Headaches

- More commonly, patients with brain tumors experience nonspecific, intermittent, tension-type headaches, which are not associated with other features of raised intracranial pressure.
- Most of these patients can be made comfortable with simple analgesics, weak narcotics, or a minor adjustment of steroid dose.
- Some patients have migraine-like headaches, although usually there are atypical features. Occipital tumors can be associated with intermittent visual symptoms (occipital seizures), thus mimicking the scotomata associated with migraine. Careful attention to the chronology and nature of symptoms generally differentiates these atypical features from true migraine with aura.

### Headache Location

- Headache location is generally ipsilateral to the tumor.
- In general, when the headache is occipital in location, the tumor usually is in the posterior fossa; and when the headache is frontal, the tumor is supratentorial.

- The preceding are generalizations and exceptions are common.
- When a patient with a supratentorial tumor develops a new occipital headache, the clinician should suspect increased intracranial pressure causing traction on the tentorium and impending herniation. Such a patient will be noted to tilt the head toward the side of the tumor and hold the back of the neck.

## Differential Diagnosis

Headaches in general oncology and neuro-oncology patients can be related to factors other than central nervous system (CNS) tumor. Table 41-1 lists medications that may cause or exacerbate headaches. Table 41-2 lists important diagnostic considerations. These medications and conditions may be the sole cause of the patient's headaches or represent contributing factors. Recognition and elimination or reduction of such exacerbating factors is an important part of management.

**Table 41-1**  Medications Used in Cancer Therapy That May Cause or Worsen Headaches

| Type of Medication | Specific Drugs |
|---|---|
| Chemotherapy agents | Corticosteroids<br>Procarbazine<br>Cytarabine<br>Retinoic acid<br>Tamoxifen |
| Antiemetics and gastrointestinal medications | Odansetron<br>Cimetidine<br>Granisetron<br>Dolasetron |
| Analgesics | Nonsteroidal anti-inflammatory drugs*<br>Narcotics (rebound headaches) |
| Immune modulating agents | Monoclonal antibodies*<br>Intravenous IgG*<br>OKT3*<br>Interferons |
| Antibiotics | Trimethoprim-sulfamethoxazole* |

*Can also cause aseptic meningitis.

**Table 41-2**   Nontumoral Causes of Headache Not to Miss

| Condition | Clinical Features | Evaluation and Treatment |
|---|---|---|
| Intracranial tumor with or without intratumoral hemorrhage | Hemorrhage into a primary or metastatic intracranial tumor causes an acute worsening of headache | CT or MRI scan of brain Neurosurgical intervention sometimes warranted |
| Hemorrhage due to thrombocytopenia | As in leukemia, chemotherapy induced thrombocytopenia, acute onset of headache | CT scan without contrast |
| Subarachnoid hemorrhage | Sudden onset of severe headache, with or without meningeal signs | CT scan without contrast Lumbar puncture Neurosurgical consultation |
| Temporal arteritis | Bitemporal headache Temporal artery tenderness Age >60 years Polymyalgia rheumatica Anemia | Erythrocyte sedimentation rate Complete blood count (anemia) Temporal artery biopsy Steroid therapy |
| Subdural hematoma | Nonspecific headache Constant History of falls | CT scan without contrast Neurosurgical consultation |
| Low-pressure headache ("post–lumbar puncture headache") | Occipital or holocranial Relieved by supine position Follows lumbar puncture, neurosurgical procedure, bone marrow harvest, trauma or may be spontaneous | Aggressive hydration Bedrest Analgesics Treat nausea Blood patch if persists or is severe May see meningeal enhancement on MRI |
| Systemic infection | Nonspecific headache | Evaluate for infection |
| Meningitis | Headache or meningeal signs With or without fever Photophobia | Lumbar puncture See Chapter 32 |
| Intracranial abscess | Headache Signs and symptoms of increased ICP Fever commonly absent Focal neurologic deficit | CT or MRI with contrast Lumbar puncture potentially dangerous and rarely diagnostic Neurosurgical consultation IV antibiotics See Chapter 32 |

*continues*

**Table 41-2**  Nontumoral Causes of Headache Not to Miss  *continued*

| Condition | Clinical Features | Evaluation and Treatment |
| --- | --- | --- |
| Vasculitis | New onset, nonspecific headaches with or without neurologic deficits | Erythrocyte sedimentation rate (but may be normal)<br>Evaluation for systemic vasculitis<br>Cerebral angiogram (may be normal)<br>Neurologic consultation |
| Sinusitis | Pain over sinuses<br>Nasal drainage<br>Pain increases when the patient bends over | CT scan of the sinuses |
| Pseudotumor cerebri (idiopathic intracranial hypertension) | Holocranial or frontal<br>Increased bending over<br>Transient visual obscurations<br>Obesity (80%)<br>Female (80%) | MRI of brain with contrast<br>Lumbar puncture (document elevated opening pressure)<br>Visual field exam and ophthamology consultation<br>Neurologic consultation |
| Posttraumatic headache | Can occur following craniotomy, trauma | Exclude other causes<br>Symptomatic treatment<br>NSAIDs (Indomethacin) |
| Hypothyroidism | Other signs and symptoms of hypothyroidism | T4, TSH |
| Cervical spine disease<br>Tumor<br>Herniated disc<br>Osteoporosis | Occipital headache<br>Radiation over head | Cervical spine plain films<br>Cervical spine MRI |
| Carbon dioxide retention (obstructive sleep apnea) | Morning headaches<br>Pulmonary disease<br>Daytime sleepiness | Arterial blood gas<br>Pulmonary evaluation |

CT, computed tomography; MRI, magnetic resonance imaging; NSAIDs, nonsteroidal anti-inflammatory drugs; TSH, thyroid-stimulating hormone.

## Management

### Brain Tumor Headaches

- Management of the tumor.
- Medication to relieve symptoms.
- Management of raised ICP and CSF obstruction, if present.
- Elevating the head of the patient's bed if increased ICP is suspected.

- Avoiding Valsalva maneuvers, including sudden position changes, vomiting, and constipation.
- Having patient learn relaxation techniques.

### *Symptomatic Headache Treatments*

Although the treatment of headaches commonly is to relieve symptoms, the clinician must first consider and exclude the important causes of headaches as listed in Table 41-2. When no specific cause is found, headaches are treated symptomatically. When nausea and vomiting are present, the addition of antiemetics (see Chapter 46) is beneficial and aids in headache control. Specific approaches to the treatment of pain, including headaches, can be found in Chapter 54.

## Suggested Reading

Forsyth PA, Posner JB. Headaches in patients with brain tumors: A study of 111 patients. *Neurology.* 1993;43(9):1678–1683.

Forsyth PA, Posner JB. Secondary headaches: Intracranial neoplasms. In J Olesen, P Tfelt-Hansen, KMA Welch (eds). *The Headaches.* New York: Raven Press, 1993:705–714.

Honig PJ, Charney EB. Children with brain tumor headaches: Distinguishing features. *Am J Dis Child.* 1982;136(2):121–124.

Ray BS, Wolff HG. Experimental studies on headache: Pain-sensitive structures of the head and their significance in headache. *Arch Surg.* 1940; 41(4):813–856.

# 42

# Hiccups

Hiccups in cancer patients are a source of distress and discomfort when they become prolonged or intractable. Occasional patients with prolonged, intractable, or recurrent hiccups will develop aspiration pneumonia or nutritional depletion. The new onset of hiccups also may herald a change in the patient's disease state. This chapter outlines the causes of hiccups and provides a practical approach to treatment.

## Terms

- Hiccup: closure of the glottis in conjunction with clonic spasm of the diaphragm and accessory muscles of inspiration; usually only the left diaphragm is involved.
- Persistent or protracted hiccups: a single episode of hiccups lasting over 48 hours.
- Intractable hiccups: a single episode of hiccups lasting over a month and refracting to interventions.

## Differential Diagnosis

### Neurologic Causes

- Increased intracranial pressure.
- Traction on tentorium due to supratentorial mass lesion.
- Vascular event or tumor of the basal ganglia or brain stem.
- Must be distinguished from palatal myoclonus, which has a faster rate (60–100 times/min vs. hiccups 4–60 times/min). In palatal myoclonus, the palate and uvula elevate repeatedly, causing a clicking noise. Palatal myoclonus may respond to clonazepam or valproic acid.

## Medication Causes

- Corticosteroids, barbiturates, and benzodiazepines are the medications that most frequently cause hiccups.
- Other possible medications include antidepressants, dopaminergic antiparkinson agents, beta-lactams, macrolides, fluoroquinolones, digitalis, opioids, and nonsteroidal anti-inflammatory drugs.
- Cancer patients may be on one or more of these medications and have other causative conditions; identifying a single causative agent in an individual patient may be impossible. However, modifying only one of many contributing factors may be sufficient to provide relief.

## Gastrointestinal

- Gastric distension, slowed gastric motility.
- Gastroesophageal reflux.

## Metabolic

- Hypocalcemia.
- Hyponatremia.
- Sepsis.
- Uremia.

## Structural

Structural causes include tumors irritating the vagus or phrenic nerves in the head and neck, lung, or mediastinum.

## Treatment

- Identify and treat the underlying conditions.
- Pharmacologic treatment is outlined in Table 42-1.

**Table 42-1**  Pharmacology and Treatment for Hiccups

| Drug | Dosing | Comments and Side Effects |
|---|---|---|
| Chlorpromazine | 25–50 mg IM, then 25–50 mg IM or PO q 8 hours | Drug of choice<br>Hypotension, sedation<br>Extrapyramidal reaction |
| Haloperidol | 2–5 mg IM, then 1–4 mg PO q 8 hours | Hypotension, sedation<br>Extrapyramidal reaction |
| Metoclopramide | Loading dose 0.5–1.0 mg IV, up to 1–2 mg/kg every 2 hours | Helpful when gastroparesis is a contributing factor<br>Akathisia and extrapyramidal reactions |
| Baclofen | 10–20 mg PO, may increase by 10 mg increments if needed | Helpful when etiology is neurologic<br>Sedation, insomnia, dizziness, weakness, ataxia, and confusion |
| Dexamethasone | For patients not on steroids, give 10–20 mg IV<br>For patients on steroids, give a bolus of 10–20 mg IV and double the maintenance dose | Helpful when increased intracranial pressure is the cause, however, some patients develop hiccups from high-dose steroids |
| Phenytoin | 200–300 mg IV (at a rate of <50 mg/min), repeat up to 15 mg/kg | |
| Midazolam | 5–10 mg bolus IV, then 40–120 mg/24 hours IV or by subcutaneous infusion | Helpful when IV access is problematic (can be infused subcutaneously)<br>Sedation, hypotension |

IM, intramuscular; PO, oral; IV, intravenous.

## Suggested Reading

Bagheri H, Cismondo S, Montastruc JL. Drug-induced hiccup: A review of the France pharmacologic vigilance database. [French] *Therapie.* 1999; 54(1):35–39.

Friedman NL. Hiccups: A treatment review. *Pharmacotherapy.* 1996;16(6): 986–995.

Johnson BR, Kriel RL. Baclofen for chronic hiccups. *Pediatr Neurol.* 1996; 15(1):66–67.

Peleg R, Shvartzman P. Hiccup. *J Fam Pract.* 1996;42(4):424.

Wilcock A, Twycross R. Midazolam for intractable hiccup. *J Pain Symptom Manage.* 1996;12(1):59–61.

# 43

# Increased Intracranial Pressure, Herniation Syndromes, and Coma

Increased intracranial pressure (ICP) and cerebral herniation syndromes are the most life-threatening emergencies occurring in brain tumor patients. Although many brain tumor patients have chronically elevated intracranial pressure that can be managed on an outpatient basis, some will present with acute or progressive increased ICP and require hospitalization and emergency management. Recognizing the presence of acutely increased ICP with impending herniation and appropriate management can be life saving and allows for further treatment of the patient's tumor. The clinician also must recognize that it is not always appropriate to aggressively treat increased ICP, such as in a patient who has failed tumor therapy and desires only supportive care.

## Mechanisms

Four general mechanisms result in increased ICP in primary brain tumor and cancer patients:

1. Brain edema, which in turn can be related to several mechanisms. Elevated ICP can be focal or diffuse and continuous or intermittent.
2. Compression or obstruction of venous outflow (intracranial sinuses, superior vena cava).
3. Ventricular obstruction (obstructive hydrocephalus).
4. Nonobstructing hydrocephalus due to impaired cerebrospinal fluid (CSF) reabsorption (usual cause) or increased production (rare).

## Presentation

Common:

- Headaches.
- Nausea or vomiting.
- Confusion.

Less common:

- Loss of balance.
- Plateau waves (see following).
- Tinnitus.

Patients harboring intracranial tumors may have compensated increased ICP and experience transient acute rises in ICP ("plateau waves" or pressure waves). These may be spontaneous but usually are precipitated by position changes, endotracheal suctioning, sneezing, coughing, or other Valsalva maneuvers. Modest rises in systemic blood pressure also can cause increased symptoms in patients with baseline elevated ICP.

## Clinical Evaluation

The following items are important to examine when evaluating the patient with suspected increased ICP. Table 43-1 categorizes types of coma by the level of involvement in the nervous system.

- Level of consciousness: Confusion → delirium → stupor → coma (see Chapter 45 for descriptions).
- Pupils: Examine the size of pupils in room lighting, response to direct light, and consensual response to light (constriction of opposite pupil).
- Oculocephalic maneuver ("doll's eyes"): Gently turn patient's head to the left and right, up and down and monitor eyes for movement. Do not attempt this maneuver if there is suspected C-spine instability. In awake patients, this test is not interpretable and causes patient distress.
  - Normal:
    Turn head to right, eyes deviate to left.
    Turn head to left, eyes deviate to right.
    Turn head downward, eyes deviate upward.
    Turn head upward, eyes deviate downward.
  - Abnormal:
    Lack of eye deviation in response to movement as just described indicates brain stem pathology.
    Normal responses to oculocephalic testing in the comatose patient suggest that the brain stem is intact and the pathology involves both cerebral hemispheres (e.g., toxic or metabolic coma).

**Table 43-1** Increased Intracranial Pressure and Herniation Syndromes: A Guide to Diagnosis

| Herniation Syndrome (structures affected) | Process | Vascular Involvement | Level of Consciousness and Clinical Signs | Pupils | Eye Movements | Respiration |
|---|---|---|---|---|---|---|
| Increased ICP with herniation (depends on site of tumor) | Focal or generalized brain edema | Intracranial venous stasis, decreased venous return | Normal to confusion or delirium Babinski: one or both | Normal and reactive | Depends on site of lesion (see Chapter 52) | Normal to tachypneic |
| Cingulate gyrus herniation (cingulate gyrus) | Cingulate gyrus under falx | Ipsilateral internal cerebral vein and anterior cerebral artery | Normal to confusion, delirium, stupor | Normal | Depends on site of lesion | Normal to tachypneic |
| Central herniation: | Bilateral hemispheric mass effect compresses diencephalon and midbrain | Traction on penetrating vessels of midbrain and pons | Coma | | | |
| Early diencephalic | | | Withdraws to stimulus, Babinski: bilateral | Small and reactive | Present | Cheyne-Stokes |
| Late diencephalic | | | Motionless, arms flexed, legs extended | Small and reactive | Present | Cheyne-Stokes |

| Site | Mechanism | Vascular | Motor/Posture | Pupils | Eye movements | Respiration |
|---|---|---|---|---|---|---|
| Midbrain or pons | | | Motionless, arms and legs extended | Dilated or midposition, fixed | Disconjugate or absent | Central neurogenic |
| Pons or medulla | | | Motionless, flaccid | Midposition, fixed | Absent | Shallow, rapid, ataxic |
| Uncal herniation: | Uncus herniates through tentorial notch, compresses midbrain and third nerve | Ipsilateral posterior cerebral artery | Coma Contralateral Babinski and increased tone | | | |
| Early third nerve | | | | Ipsilateral pupil sluggish, midposition to dilated | Present or disconjugate | Normal |
| Late third nerve (then follows central herniation pattern) | | | | Ipsilateral fixed and dilated | Incomplete | Hyperventilation |
| Foramen magnum herniation (medulla and lower cranial nerves) | Posterior fossa mass effect pushes tonsils through foramen magnum | | Coma to brain death | Bilateral fixed and dilated | Motionless, flaccid | Agonal to none |

- Oculovestibular testing by caloric stimulation: This test should only be performed if the oculocephalic test is negative and the patient is comatose (no eye deviation in response to movement).
    - Elevate head of bed 30 degrees.
    - Examine external auditory canal to confirm the integrity of the tympanic membrane and that the canal is clear of debris and wax.
    - Irrigate ear with ice water using small, blunt tipped catheter gently placed in external canal.
    - The patient's eyes should slowly deviate conjugately to irrigated ear. If the patient is not in deep coma, there may be a corrective fast (nystagmus) movement away from irrigated ear.
    - A normal response demonstrates that the pons and midbrain are intact. An abnormal response may indicate focal pathology (e.g., a unilateral CN VI palsy) or diffuse pathology (e.g., severe metabolic depression).

## Management

### Acute Increased Intracranial Pressure

The first step is to decide whether the patient warrants aggressive inpatient management. This is indicated when

- There is a progressive course of signs and symptoms of increased ICP and threat of cerebral herniation as described previously.
- There are reasonable treatment options to offer the patient.
- The patient has not refused aggressive management. Aggressive management is not always appropriate. However, palliative measures can and should be implemented even when vigorous intervention is not warranted. Both the status of the tumor and the patient's directives must be taken into account.

A raised ICP with threatened herniation is a neurologic emergency and warrants admission to the intensive care unit. Table 43-2 summarizes the approach to the control of increased ICP. Clinicians who are not experienced in the management of these patients should quickly obtain consultation for assistance. Refer to the Suggested Reading section for more detailed discussions of management. Tumor-related edema can require very large doses of steroids. Dexamethasone "loading" doses of 50–100 mg and daily doses of 40–80 mg are needed for large tumors with significant mass effect. Intubation can cause transient but severe increases in ICP, particularly in partially awake patients. Premedication or sedation is critical. Some patients with raised ICP spontaneously hyperventilate but intubation still is needed to control the airway and avoid aspiration. Lumbar puncture is contraindicated in all patients with uncontrolled increased ICP.

**Table 43-2**  Guidelines for the Inpatient Management of Adults with Acute
Raised Intracranial Pressure

| Intervention | Specifics | Mechanism | Comments |
|---|---|---|---|
| Hyperventilation | Intubation and hyperventilation aiming for $pCO_2$ of 25–30 mmHg | Lowers $pCO_2$ | Immediately effective<br>ICP may "rebound" in a few hours<br>Follow ABGs, electrolytes<br>Further decrease of $pCO_2$ is not helpful |
| Mannitol | Loading dose 1–2 g/kg IV, then 0.5–1.0 g/kg as needed to control ICP | Decreases brain edema | Onset after several minutes<br>Transiently effective<br>May see "rebound" after 24–48 hours<br>Follow electrolytes and fluid status, serum osmolarity |
| Dexamethasone | Loading dose 10–100 mg IV<br>Maintenance dose 6–20 mg IV q 4–6 hours | Tightens blood/brain barrier | Peak effect several hours after first dose but is durable<br>Follow electrolytes, glucose, anticonvulsant levels, consider H-2 blocker |
| Neurosurgical interventions:<br>ICP monitoring | ICP monitoring assists use of preceding techniques | | |
| Ventricular drainage | Ventricular drainage in cases of obstruction | Relieves obstruction | Posterior fossa and intraventricular tumors |
| Tumor decompression | Tumor decompression when patient is stabilized | Decreases mass effect of tumor | |
| Diuretics | Furosamide 10–40 mg IV, then as needed to control fluid status | Diuretic | Poor evidence to support this treatment<br>Intravascular depletion |

*continues*

**Table 43-2**   Guidelines for the Inpatient Management of Adults with Acute Raised Intracranial Pressure   *continued*

| Intervention | Specifics | Mechanism | Comments |
|---|---|---|---|
| Fluid management | Avoid fluid overload<br>Avoid hypotonic fluids and sudden shifts of blood volume | Avoid increased brain edema<br>Avoid hyponatremia, which can cause seizures and increased ICP | |
| General care | Elevate head of bed<br>Avoid Valsalva maneuver<br>Avoid agitation<br>Prevent seizures | Avoid sudden increases in ICP | Premedicate for procedures<br>Sedate if needed |
| Blood pressure | Avoid raised SBP<br>Monitor SBP and MAP | | |

ABGs, arterial blood gases; SBP, systolic blood pressure; MAP, mean arterial pressure.

## Chronic Increased Intracranial Pressure

The management of chronically raised ICP, summarized in Table 43-3, is part of appropriate palliative care of the brain tumor patient. Treatment should be aimed at controlling the patient's symptoms and preserving the quality of life rather than at other artificial "endpoints," such as the results of magnetic resonance imaging (MRI) scans or presence of papilledema. Patients who do not tolerate corticosteroids generally can be managed by decreasing the steroid doses and treating specific symptoms. Simple measures, such as elevating the head of the bed at home to minimize nocturnal and morning headaches, can significantly improve the quality of life. Lumbar puncture is contraindicated and may cause brain herniation.

**Table 43-3**  Guidelines for the Management of Adult Outpatients with Chronically Raised Intracranial Pressure

| Intervention | Specifics | Mechanism | Comments |
|---|---|---|---|
| Dexamethasone | Loading dose of 6–10 mg, then daily dose of 8–40 mg in divided doses | Tightens blood/brain barrier | Follow glucose Fluid status Balance side effects vs. desired effects Minimize dose as possible See Chapter 14 |
| Control headache | Narcotics usually are needed May respond to increased steroid dose See Chapter 41 | Symptomatic | |
| Control nausea | See Chapter 46 | Vomiting increases ICP | |
| Control seizures | See Chapter 50 | Seizures may acutely raise ICP | |
| Avoid hypercarbia | Treat sleep apnea, obstructive pulmonary disease | Lower $pCO_2$ | |
| Elevate head of bed | 30–45° | Lowers ICP | Hospital bed Foam wedge Helps alleviate nocturnal and A.M. headaches |
| Avoid Valsalva maneuver | Prophylaxis for constipation Use cough suppressants Avoid sudden movements or bending | Prevent sudden rises in ICP | |
| Follow optic nerve function | Ophthamologic follow-up, visual fields | Chronic ICP can cause visual loss | Not always preventable |

## Suggested Reading

Abdelwahab W, Frishman W, Landau A. Management of hypertensive urgencies and emergencies. *J Clin Pharmacol.* 1995;35(8):747–762.

Plum F, Posner JB. *The Diagnosis of Stupor and Coma* (3rd ed). Philadelphia: F.A. Davis, 1980.

Ropper AH. *Neurologic and Neurosurgical Intensive Care* (3rd ed). New York: Raven Press, 1993.

# 44

# Insomnia

Changes in sleep pattern are frequent symptoms in cancer patients and may cause emotional distress and loss of a patient's sense of well-being. Insomnia can exacerbate other, ongoing symptoms, particularly pain. Insomnia is characterized by one or more of the following components: difficulty falling asleep, difficulty remaining asleep, early morning waking, or awakening not feeling rested (nonrestorative sleep). Successful management includes both pharmacologic and behavioral approaches.

## Contributing Factors

- Depression or other psychological manifestations of illness.
- Anxiety or emotional distress regarding the tumor, treatment, existential issues, death, or personal or family problems.
- Pain, which in turn can increase in intensity due to sleep deprivation.
- Certain medications: corticosteroids, caffeine, and alcohol.
- Nocturnal seizures.
- Nausea or vomiting.
- Dyspnea, coughing.
- Incontinence.
- Spasticity.
- Nocturnal headaches.
- Hospitalization, scheduled medications.
- Fear of falling asleep and not waking up.

## Assessment of Insomnia

Sleep patterns vary a great deal among individuals. What is important to the patient is the perception of insomnia and whether the patient feels rested. Key questions to ask the patient include

- Do you feel you are sleeping well? Did you feel you were sleeping well before your tumor diagnosis?
- Do you feel rested in the morning?
- Have your sleep patterns changed since your diagnosis? How? Are you having trouble falling asleep, staying asleep, waking up too early, or having unpleasant dreams?
- Do you find that you are sleepy during the day? How much are you napping during the day?
- Do you use alcoholic drinks, coffee or tea, tobacco? How much? When?
- What do you think is preventing you from sleeping well?

## Nonmedication Management

- Patients may need help defining and accepting new sleep patterns. The patient's previous sleep pattern or generally accepted sleep pattern may no longer be feasible.
- Provide ideas about how to fill, and even enjoy, the time spent awake at night.
- Physician and other appointments and other activities of daily living often can be scheduled early or late in the day to accommodate patients' patterns.
- Limit daytime naps as feasible.
- Institute a predictable bedtime routine and time.
- Have the patient remain out of bed during the daytime, even if just to another place to rest, so that the bed and bedroom are associated with sleep.
- Suggest warm milk, selected herbal and decaffeinated teas, carbohydrate snack at bedtime.
- Suggest warm bath, massage, sexual activity for inducing relaxation.
- Assess home environment (lighting, temperature, ventilation, noise level) to maximize relaxing setting for the patient.
- Elevate head of bed for respiratory distress or headaches caused by intracranial pressure.
- Suggest use of radio, television, books to stimulate sleepiness.
- Suggest use of biofeedback and other behavior modification therapies.
- Pain medications may need to be increased at night.

- Make bathroom facilities easily accessible during the night to minimize the disturbance of nocturia: bedside commode, handheld urinal.
- Schedule diuretics and laxatives in the morning.
- Schedule stimulating medications early in the day.

## Suggested Reading

Sateia MJ, Silberfarb PM. Sleep in palliative care. In D Doyle, GWC Hanks, N MacDonald (eds). *Oxford Textbook of Palliative Medicine.* Oxford, England: Oxford University Press, 1995.

Waller A, Caroline NL. *Handbook of Palliative Care in Cancer* (2nd ed). Boston: Butterworth–Heinemann, 2000.

# 45

# Mental Status Changes

Mental status changes are a common complication in cancer patients, present in about 12% of oncology hospital admissions. Mental status changes can occur from focal or diffuse neurologic processes or medical conditions. Many of these conditions are readily treatable, such as hypoglycemia, and others can be managed to reduce symptoms and optimize neurologic function. Some situations are part of an end stage of the patient's cancer. For these patients, recognition of encephalopathy guides appropriate management.

## Classification

Mental status changes occur along a spectrum that reflects level of consciousness:

confusion → delirium → stupor → coma

where

*Confusion* is the impaired ability to think in the usual manner, including attention deficits, slow processing, altered perception of the environment (illusions, delusions, hallucinations), or altered sense of time and place. Symptoms may fluctuate and there may be lucid periods.

*Delirium* includes features of confusion with impaired attention. Other features include alterations of sleep/wake cycle, agitation, and heightened arousal.

*Stupor* involves decreased alertness, decreased arousal, minimal spontaneous motor activity, and slowed responses.

*Coma* is the state of unarousable unresponsiveness. There is no spontaneous motor behavior and respirations usually are abnormal.

## Causes of Change in Mental Status

### Metabolic

- Hyponatremia.
- Hypoglycemia.
- Hypercarbia.
- Hypercalcemia.
- Hypoxia.
- Hepatic encephalopathy.
- Renal failure.
- Disseminated intravascular coagulation.
- Thiamin deficiency.
- Pancreatitis.
- Postoperative or intensive care unit (ICU) psychosis (diagnosis of exclusion).
- Hyperthyroidism (rare).

### Toxic Encephalopathy

- Anticonvulsant agents:
  - Valproate.
  - Phenytoin.
  - Phenobarbital.
  - Carbamazepine.
  - Levateracitam.
  - Topirimate.
- Chemotherapy agents:
  - Procarbazine: encephalopathy, headaches, reverses with removal of drug.
  - L-asparaginase: sinus thrombosis or strokes.
  - Methotrexate: intrathecal or high-dose IV.
  - Cytarabine: especially high dose.
  - 5-FU/Levamisole.
  - Cyclosporine.
  - Interleukin-2.
  - Ifosphamide: 20–30% of patients develop acute encephalopathy with cerebellar signs, hallucinations, and seizures. Risk factors include impaired renal function, dose, low serum albumin, and older age. The condition reverses with cessation of treatment.

- – Tamoxifen: high dose.
- – Cisplatin: direct neurotoxicity rare with IV use, symptoms more often relate to hydration (water intoxication) or associated nephrotoxicity (hypomagnesemia or hypocalcemia).
- Intrathecal drugs.
- Non-chemotherapy-drug overdoses such as anticholinergics, amphetamines, corticosteroids, benzodiazepines, and opiates.
- Drug withdrawal: narcotics, barbiturates, and antidepressant agents.
- Alcohol withdrawal, including delirium tremens.
- Neuroleptic malignant syndrome: dopamine antagonists such as haloperidol.

## Tumor

- Brain metastases.
- Leptomeningeal metastases.
- Hydrocephalus.
- Paraneoplastic encephalopathy.

## Infection (see Chapter 32)

- Encephalitis: viral (herpes, cytomegalovirus, varicella zoster).
- Meningitis: bacterial, fungal.
- Brain abscess: toxoplasmosis, bacterial, fungal.
- Systemic infection: sepsis.

## Radiation Encephalopathy

- Acute: during radiotherapy.
- Early delayed: 2 months after radiotherapy.
- Late.

## Vascular Disease

- Stroke.
- Nonbacterial thrombotic endocarditis or disseminated intravascular coagulation.
- Subdural hematoma.
- Subarachnoid hemorrhage.
- Hypertensive encephalopathy.
- Vasculitis.
- Pulmonary emboli.
- Transient global amnesia.

## Epileptic

- Postictal confusion: consider unwitnessed seizure.
- Nonconvulsive status epilepticus.

## Psychiatric

- Depression and anxiety (see Chapter 36).
- Schizophrenia.
- Bipolar disorder.

# Approach and Treatment

## Initial Management

- *Acute treatment:* begin during initial diagnostic process in patients with stupor or coma.
  - "ABCs": ensure adequate airway, breathing, and circulation.
  - Obtain IV access.
  - Pulse oximetry: apply oxygen if hypoxic.
  - IV thiamine 100 mg.
  - Intravenous dextrose: 50 ml of D50W (if glucose level is low or unobtainable).
  - For suspected narcotic overdose: Naloxone (Narcan): 0.4–1.2 mg IV.
  - For suspected benzodiazepine overdose: Flumazenil 0.2 mg IV over 30 seconds, 0.3 mg 1 minute later, then 0.5 mg every minute for a total dose of 3 mg.
  - *STAT labs:* complete blood count (CBC), electrolytes, blood glucose, BUN/creatinine, arterial blood gases, toxicology screen and anticonvulsant levels.

## History

Obtain information on the nature and extent of tumor, recent therapies, oral intake, comorbidities, medication use, history of seizures, recent falls, and advanced directives.

## Examination

- General medical:
  - Nuchal rigidity.
  - Papilledema.
  - Evidence of trauma.

– Evidence of infection.
– Autonomic signs.
- Neurologic (see Chapter 43 for the coma examination):
  – State of arousal.
  – Thought processes, attention, orientation.
  – Focal neurologic deficits such as aphasia, amnesia, neglect, and visual field deficits.
  – Asterixis, myoclonus.
  – Reflexes.
  – Plantar responses.

## Laboratory Tests

- Initial STAT tests, as previously.
- Transaminases (AST, ALT), ammonia, serum albumin.
- T4, thyroid-stimulating hormone.
- Chest X ray.
- Electrocardiogram.
- Neuro-imaging.
- Lumbar puncture, if indicated.
- Electroencephalogram, if indicated.

## Management

- Consider ICU care.
- Treat underlying disorders.
- Evaluate medication usage: eliminate or reduce sedatives, anticholinergics.
- Environment: quiet, dim light at night, familiar visitors, familiar objects.
- Avoid sensory deprivation or overstimulation.
- An attendant often is needed for agitated or confused patients.
- Advanced directives (patient's desires for aggressive care) should be considered if this information is available.

## Suggested Reading

Plum F, Posner JB. *The Diagnosis of Stupor and Coma* (3rd ed). Philadelphia: F.A. Davis, 1982.

Posner JB. *Neurologic Complications of Cancer.* Philadelphia: F.A. Davis, 1995.

# 46

# Nausea and Vomiting

Chemotherapy is an effective treatment for many neoplasms. Still, the toxicity of therapy can be daunting to physicians and frightening to patients. Nausea and vomiting are the most troublesome side effects of chemotherapy to patients and can be severe enough that some patients forego useful therapy. Fortunately, the serotonin receptor antagonists have revolutionized the control of chemotherapy-induced nausea and vomiting.

It is critical to control acute treatment-related nausea and vomiting from the onset of therapy, as failure to do so may predispose patients to anticipatory nausea with later treatment cycles. Some patients experience little or no acute nausea but are plagued by a syndrome of delayed nausea, which requires specific attention. Table 46-1 provides medication management for nausea and vomiting.

## Mechanisms

Although the mechanism of nausea and vomiting is not fully understood, several things are known. There are thought to be two different general mechanisms: a peripheral reflex and a centrally mediated reflex. Serotonin (5-hydroxytryptamine) is an important messenger in these pathways, and medications that block a subset of serotonin receptors (the 5-HT$_3$ receptors or serotonin type 3 receptors) are critical in controlling chemotherapy-induced nausea.

Distention or perturbation of the gastrointestinal tract can stimulate a release of serotonin from enterochromaffin cells, which contain the majority of the body's serotonin. This mediates stimulation of the nucleus of the solitary tract via the vagus nerve, which in turn activates the "vomiting center." When the vomiting center is ablated in animal models, nausea and vomiting

**Table 46-1**  Medications Helpful for Treating Nausea and Vomiting

| Situation | Regimen | Comments and Considerations |
|---|---|---|
| Prevention of nausea and vomiting | Granisetron 1 mg IV or PO<br>Dexamethasone 10 mg IV or PO<br>*or*<br>Ondansetron 8 mg IV or PO<br>Dexamethasone 10 mg IV or PO<br>*or*<br>Dolasteron 100 mg PO<br>Dexamethasone 10 mg IV or PO<br>*or*<br>Granisetron 2 mg PO<br>Dexamethasone* 10 mg IV or PO | To be used with moderate to highly emetogenic regimens |
| | Droperidol, 1.25–2.5 mg IV<br>*or*<br>Prochlorperazine, 10 mg PO | To be used with agents of low emetogenic potential |
| Delayed nausea and vomiting | Dexamethasone* 8 mg PO bid or 4 doses, then Dexamethasone* 4 mg PO bid for 4 doses<br>*and*<br>Metoclopramide 30 mg PO q6h for 16 doses | Consider in patients with nausea and vomiting, clinical history of delayed nausea and vomiting, or in those receiving ≥100 mg/m² of cisplatin |
| Anticipatory nausea and vomiting | Lorazepam 0.5–2.0 mg SL or PO 1–2 hours before treatment; may give earlier PRN | |
| Nausea during radiation | Metoclopramide 10–30 mg PO q6h | |
| Nausea due to increased intracranial pressure | Dexamethasone 4 mg PO q6h<br>Elevate head of bed 30–40° | |

IV, intravenous; PO, oral; SL, sublingual; PRN, as needed.

*Use if other agents fail or increased intracranial pressure is suspected.

are prevented. Peripheral mechanisms appear to be the most important in cisplatin-induced nausea and vomiting.

An area outside the blood/brain barrier, termed the *chemoreceptor trigger zone* (CTZ), is found in the brain stem in the postrema area. When exposed to certain chemical stimuli (such as emetogenic chemotherapy agents) in the cerebrospinal fluid or blood, the vomiting center can be activated. This area of the brain has receptors for dopamine, serotonin, and opiates.

## Anticipatory Nausea

Anticipatory nausea is a learned response, and its prevalence seems to have decreased with the widespread use of serotonin receptor antagonists. However, it remains a vexing problem for some patients. When this problem requires intervention, oral or sublingual lorazepam in a dose of 0.5–1.0 mg 2–4 hours before the scheduled treatment may be useful. This agent is a moderately effective antiemetic, which also has amnesic and anxiolytic effects (Laszlo et al., 1985).

## Acute Nausea

Serotonin receptor antagonists are the standard to prevent acute chemotherapy-related nausea. The currently available agents are ondansetron, granisetron, and dolasetron. Well-controlled trials document that emesis can be prevented in the majority of patients receiving moderately emetogenic chemotherapy. Furthermore, this control is achieved without sedation and without extrapyramidal side effects. The efficacy of these agents is enhanced by the addition of corticosteroids such as dexamethasone (Italian Group for Antiemetic Research, 1995).

## Delayed Nausea

While the serotonin receptor antagonists are effective in *preventing* nausea and vomiting, they are less successful in established nausea. Also, chemotherapy may lead to a syndrome of delayed nausea and vomiting, particularly when agents such as cisplatin are part of the regimen. In individuals who have delayed nausea and vomiting, the use of dexamethasone and metoclopramide results in improved control (Kris et al., 1989). This approach includes dexamethasone, 8 mg PO bid for 2 days followed by 4 mg bid for 2 additional days combined with metoclopramide, 0.5 mg/kg (usually 30 mg) PO qid for 4 days.

## Other Causes of Nausea and Vomiting

Nausea and vomiting in brain tumor patients not always is due to chemotherapy. Persistent nausea not temporally related to chemotherapy should alert the physician to other possibilities. In patients with brain cancer, increased intracranial pressure can be a prominent cause. Early intervention with steroids may yield dramatic improvement. Side effects from nonchemotherapy drugs also may be related to nausea. Aggressive pain control often requires narcotics, commonly associated with nausea. Alteration in the medication or route of administration may assist in alleviating this problem.

Other etiologies may include hypercalcemia, bowel obstruction, or uremia. As medications are a frequent cause, all prescriptions should be carefully reviewed.

## References

Italian Group for Antiemetic Research. Dexamethasone, granisetron, or both for the prevention of nausea and vomiting during chemotherapy for cancer. *N Engl J Med*. January 1995;332(1): 1–5.

Kris MG, Gralla RJ, Tyson LB, et al. Controlling delayed vomiting: Double-blind, randomized trial comparing placebo, dexamethasone alone, and metoclopramide plus dexamethasone in patients receiving cisplatin. *J Clin Oncol*. January 1989;7(1):108–114.

Laszlo J, Clark RA, Hanson DC, et al. Lorazepam in cancer patients treated with cisplatin: A drug having antiemetic, amnesic, and anxiolytic effects. *J Clin Oncol*. June 1985;3(6):864–869.

# 47

# Paraneoplastic Syndromes

Paraneoplastic neurologic syndromes (PNS) are degenerative disorders of the nervous system that occur in association with a systemic neoplasm but are not due to direct invasion of the nervous system by tumor. PNS can involve the central or the peripheral nervous system and can occur during the patient's illness with cancer, during apparent remission, or can precede the diagnosis of cancer. Antibody associations have been described for some but not all of the PNS (Table 47-1). Autoimmune mechanisms have been postulated but not proven in the pathogenesis of these conditions. The diagnosis of PNS allows appropriate patient counseling and, in some cases, may predict the presence of a neoplasm. With few exceptions, treatment is supportive.

## Overview

PNS are uncommon but important explanations for neurologic syndromes in cancer patients. Certain clinical features suggest the presence of a PNS:

- Most PNS, other than neuropathies, cause *severe*, irreversible neurologic deficits.
- The *onset of symptoms is subacute*. Patients with acute, chronic, or relapsing/remitting conditions are unlikely to have PNS. Paraneoplastic cerebellar degeneration has very rapid onset, with deficits developing over a few days.
- Most PNS are *painless* with the exception of sensory neuronopathy and dermatomyositis.

**Table 47-1**    Paraneoplastic Neurologic Syndromes, Antibody and Tumor
Associations

| Syndrome | Antibody | Most Frequently Associated Tumors |
|---|---|---|
| Subacute cerebellar degeneration | Anti-Yo | Ovarian cancer Breast cancer |
| | Anti-Hu (encephalomyelitis) | Small-cell lung cancer |
| | Anti-Ri | Breast cancer |
| | Anti-Tr | Hodgkin's lymphoma |
| Opsoclonus-myoclonus-ataxia | Anti-Ri | Breast cancer Neuroblastoma (childhood) |
| Encephalomyelitis | Anti-Hu | Small-cell lung cancer |
| Limbic encephalitis | Anti-Hu | Small-cell lung cancer |
| Limbic encephalitis | Anti-Ma Ta | Testicular cancer |
| Cancer-associated retinopathy | Anti-Hu | Small-cell lung cancer Melanoma Gynecologic tumors |
| Subacute sensory neuropathy | Anti-Hu | Small-cell lung cancer |
| Subacute motor neuronopathy | Not identified | Hodgkin's or non-Hodgkin's lymphoma |
| Lambert-Eaton myasthenic syndrome | Antibodies to presynaptic calcium channels of motor neurons | Small-cell lung cancer |

- Most patients have signs and symptoms relative to one anatomic region of the nervous system. The exception to this is patients with anti-Hu-associated encephalomyelitis, who develop symptoms relative to two or more areas of the nervous system.

## Syndromes and Classification

### Paraneoplastic Cerebellar Degeneration

Paraneoplastic cerebellar degeneration (PCD) presents with sub-acute onset of vertigo, imbalance, dysequilibrium, diplopia, or nausea and vomiting followed by the rapid development of truncal and appendicular ataxia, tremor, and dysarthria. Many patients have antibodies to cerebellar Purkinje cells (designated as anti-Yo or anti-Purkinje cell antibodies) and a gynecologic cancer. About two thirds of such patients have the onset of neurologic symptoms prior to the diagnosis of their tumor. Patients with signs and symptoms relative to other parts of the nervous system, in addition to cerebellar symptoms, generally have tumors other than gynecologic cancer and some have other antibodies (designated as anti-Hu or anti-Ri). About 50% of adults with subacute cerebellar degeneration have PNS.

### Encephalomyelitis

Encephalomyelitis is characterized by dysfunction at more than one level of the nervous system and may occur in the setting of a known neoplasm or predate the diagnosis of cancer. The most common tumor associated with encephalomyelitis is small-cell lung cancer and most patients have anti-Hu antibodies. A variety of associated tumors have been reported. Symptoms are subacute and progressive in onset and may include

- Myelitis: subacute, progressive weakness and posterior column dysfunction; both lower and upper motor neuron signs may be seen.
- Limbic encephalitis: dysfunction of the limbic system with confusion, anxiety, depression, memory loss, seizures, emotional lability, and hallucinations.
- Cerebellar degeneration: acute to subacute onset of dizziness, dysarthria, vertigo, ataxia, nausea, coarse tremor, and nystagmus. If associated with other features of encephalomyelitis, the anti-Hu antibody often is found and is strongly suggestive of small-cell lung cancer. If associated with breast cancer or gynecologic malignancies, the anti-Yo antibody may be found.
- Sensory neuronopathy (dorsal root ganglionitis): subacute sensory loss and dysesthetic pain is followed by sensory ataxia. This syndrome typically precedes tumor diagnosis but only 20% of all patients with sensory neuronopathy have a PNS.
- Bulbar encephalitis: rare as an isolated syndrome but may be associated with other features of encephalomyelitis. Patients present with lower brain stem palsies, eye movement abnormalities, vertigo, nystagmus, vomiting, and upper motor neuron signs.
- Autonomic neuropathy: gastrointestinal dysmotility, pupillary abnormalities, neurogenic bladder, and postural hypotension.

### Opsoclonus-Myoclonus-Ataxia

Patients present with opsoclonus, myoclonus, ataxia, vertigo, nausea, dysarthria, and dizziness. Some patients have anti-Ri antibodies and most of these patients have breast cancer. In children, this syndrome is associated with neuroblastoma.

## Subacute Motor Neuronopathy

Patients present with subacute bilateral weakness of the legs and upper extremities that is painless and not associated with sensory loss. Lower motor neuron signs are present.

## Lambert-Eaton Myasthenic Syndrome

Lambert-Eaton myasthenic syndrome (LEMS) presents with weakness and difficulty ambulating that improves with effort. Reflexes are hypoactive and some patients have autonomic insufficiency. Of patients with LEMS, 60–70% have cancer, usually small-cell lung cancer. The pathogenesis relates to antibody-induced impairment of acetylcholine release from presynaptic motor neurons.

## Retinal Degeneration

Patients characteristically develop progressive decline in visual acuity without pain, marked difficulty seeing in the dark, and loss of color perception. Although this may begin in one eye, it quickly involves both eyes. Some patients with paraneoplastic retinal degeneration have anti-cancer-associated retinopathy (anti-CAR) antibodies and the syndrome is associated with small-cell lung cancer, melanoma, and occasionally gynecologic malignancies.

## Limbic Encephalitis or Eye Movement Abnormalities and Testicular Cancer

This recently described PNS presents with limbic encephalitis or eye movement abnormalities and is associated with a newly characterized antibody (anti-Ma Ta). Testicular cancer is associated with this particular syndrome and antibody profile.

## Approach to the Patient

Because PNS are rare, consultation with a neurologist knowledgeable in PNS is invaluable. Other neurologic conditions should be carefully excluded. Identification of a particular antibody guides the search for a specific cancer. For example, a woman presenting with subacute cerebellar degeneration and the anti-Yo antibody is most likely to harbor a gynecologic malignancy. In patients with known cancer, other cancer-related disorders, such as metastatic tumor, infection, and toxicity due to radiotherapy or chemotherapy, are far more likely to be excluded. Evaluations may include neuro-imaging studies, cerebrospinal fluid (CSF) examination, and electrodiagnostic studies. Serum and CSF are tested for the presence of antibodies based on the clinical characterizations just described, and the CSF is tested for cell count, protein, glucose, and cytology.

With the exceptions listed here, treatment for PNS has been unrewarding. Occasional patients have responded to immunosuppression, plasmapheresis, removal of the tumor, or specific anticancer treatment:

- Opsoclonus-myoclonus syndrome may improve with treatment of the tumor, the use of clonazepam, or spontaneously.
- LEMS usually responds to immunosuppression or plasmapheresis.
- Anti-CAR retinopathy may respond to steroids.

## Suggested Reading

Bennett JL, Galetta SL, Frohman LP, et al. Neuro-ophthalmologic manifestations of a paraneoplastic syndrome and testicular carcinoma. *Neurology.* 1999;52(4):864–867.

Dalmau JO, Posner JB. Paraneoplastic syndromes. *Arch Neurol.* 1999;56(4): 405–408.

Graus F, Dalmau J, Valldeoriola F, et al. Immunological characterization of a neuronal antibody (anti-Tr) associated with paraneoplastic cerebellar degeneration and Hodgkin's disease. *J Neuroimmunology.* 1997;74(1–2): 55–61.

Jaeckle KA. Autoimmunity in paraneoplastic neurologic syndromes: Closer to the truth? *Ann Neurol.* 1999;45(2):143–145.

Jaeckle KA. Paraneoplastic nervous system syndromes. *Curr Opin Oncol.* 1996;8(3):204–208.

# 48

# Peripheral Nerve Problems: Plexopathies and Neuropathies

Peripheral nerve problems are common in cancer patients and may relate to direct tumor invasion or compression, treatment toxicity, paraneoplastic syndromes, or causes unrelated to cancer. As with other neurologic complications of cancer, accurate diagnosis guides appropriate treatment. Sensorimotor polyneuropathies are the most frequently encountered peripheral nerve syndromes. This chapter provides a general approach to peripheral nerve problems in cancer patients. The approach should enable the clinician to identify the type of peripheral nerve problem, distinguish it from peripheral nerve problems due to spinal or cerebral pathology, and guide evaluation and treatment. Pharmacologic approaches to neuropathic pain are covered in Chapter 54; the Suggested Reading section of the chapter provides more detailed information.

## Overview

Table 48-1 provides an overview of the syndromes affecting the peripheral nerves and their clinical characteristics. Table 48-2 provides a listing of peripheral nerves, muscles innervated, and their actions. Typical symptoms of peripheral nerve pathology include distal weakness and sensory changes. Weakness due to peripheral nerve pathology must be distinguished from weakness due to myopathy, neuromuscular junction (NMJ) disease, or upper motor neuron weakness. Similarly, the sensory changes encountered with peripheral nerve pathology must be distinguished from sensory deficits due to spinal cord lesions or intracranial disease. The following generalizations are helpful.

**Table 48-1**  Clinical Characteristics of Syndromes Involving the Peripheral Nerves

| Syndrome | Brief Description | Sensory Deficits | Motor Deficits | Reflexes |
|---|---|---|---|---|
| Peripheral neuropathy, sensory | Diffuse neuropathy affecting sensory nerves | Symmetric: stocking-glove pattern | None | Diminished to absent (lost early in course) Diminished distal > proximal |
| Peripheral neuropathy, motor | Diffuse neuropathy affecting motor nerves | None | Symmetric weakness: distal > proximal | Diminished to absent Diminished distal > proximal |
| Peripheral neuropathy, sensorimotor | Diffuse neuropathy affecting both sensory and motor nerves | Stocking-glove pattern | Symmetric weakness: distal > proximal | Diminished to absent (lost early in course) Diminished distal > proximal |
| Mononeuropathy | Focal neuropathy affecting one peripheral nerve (e.g., median nerve at the wrist = carpal tunnel syndrome) | Sensory loss in distribution of sensory fibers for the peripheral nerve[a] | Weakness of muscles innervated by a single peripheral nerve | Usually normal |
| Multiple mononeuropathies (mononeuritis multiplex) | Neuropathy affecting more than one peripheral nerve (e.g., median and femoral) | Sensory loss in distribution of sensory fibers for more than one peripheral nerve | Weakness of muscles innervated by more than one peripheral nerve | Normal or diminished focally |
| Radiculopathy | Neuropathy due to lesion of the nerve root as it exits the spinal column | Sensory loss in dermatome relative to the affected nerve root | Weakness of muscles in myotome relative to the affected nerve root | Diminished in radicular pattern (e.g., in C-5 radiculopathy, the bicep reflex is lost, other reflexes are normal) |
| Plexopathy[b] | Condition affecting one of the nerve plexuses (e.g., brachial, lumbar plexuses) | Sensory loss in one extremity[c] and involves more than one dermatome | Weakness of a single extremity involving mutiple nerve roots | Normal to diminished (see text) |

[a]Some peripheral nerves have no sensory fibers.    [b]Plexopathies usually are unilateral.

[c]Involves entire extremity if the entire plexus is involved, part of the extremity if only part of the plexus is involved.

**Table 48-2** Selected Peripheral Nerves and Muscles, Their Functions and Spinal Roots

| Peripheral Nerve | Muscles Innervated | Major Function | Spinal Roots[a] |
|---|---|---|---|
| **Upper extremity branches directly off the brachial plexus:** | | | |
| Dorsal scapular nerve | Rhomboids | Stabilizes scapula | C4,C5 |
| Long thoracic nerve | Serratus anterior | Stabilizes scapula | C5,C6,C7 |
| Suprascapular nerve | Supraspinatus | Abducts arm | **C5**, C6 |
| | Infraspinatus | External rotation arm | **C5**, C6 |
| Thoracodorsal nerve | Latissimus dorsi | Adducts arm | C6, **C7**, C8 |
| Pectoral nerves | Pectoralis major | Adducts arm | C5, C6, C7, C8 |
| Subscapular nerves | Teres major | Adducts arm | C5,C6,C7 |
| Spinal accessory nerve | Trapezius | Elevates shoulder | C3,C4 |
| Axillary nerve | Deltoid | Abducts arm | **C5**, C6 |
| Radial nerve | Triceps | Extension at elbow | C6, **C7**, C8 |
| | Brachioradialis | Flexion of forearm[b] | C5, **C6** |
| | Ext carpi radialis l. | Extends and abducts hand at wrist | C5, **C6** |
| Posterior interosseus nerve (terminal motor branch of radial nerve) | Supinator | Supinate forearm | C6,C7 |
| | Ext carpi ulnaris | Extends and adducts hand at wrist | **C7**, C8 |
| | Ext digitorum | Extension at meta-carpal | **C7**, C8 |
| Musculocutaneous nerve | Biceps | Flexion of arm[c] | C5, C6 |
| Median nerve, proximal to wrist | Pronator teres | Pronates forearm | C6, C7 |
| | Fl carpi radialis | Flexion and abduction of wrist | C6, C7 |
| | Fl dig prof I and II | Flexion of distal phalanges | C7, **C8** |
| | Fl pol l. | Flexion of distal phalanx of thumb | C7, **C8** |
| Median nerve, distal to wrist | Abductor pol br | Abducts thumb | C8, **T1** |
| | Opponens pol | Opposes thumb | C8, **T1** |
| Ulnar nerve, proximal to wrist | Fl carpi ulnaris | Flexion and adduction of wrist | C7, **C8**, T1 |
| | Fl dig prof III and IV | Flexion of DIP joint | C7, **C8** |

*continues*

**Table 48-2** Selected Peripheral Nerves and Muscles, Their Functions and Spinal Roots *continued*

| Peripheral Nerve | Muscles Innervated | Major Function | Spinal Roots[a] |
|---|---|---|---|
| Ulnar nerve, distal to wrist | Hypothenar muscles | Moves fifth digit | C8, **T1** |
| | Adductor pol | Adducts thumb to palm | C8, **T1** |
| | First dorsal inter-osseus | Abducts index finger | C8, **T1** |
| | Lumbricals III and IV | Adducts fingers | C8, **T1** |
| **Lower extremity:** | | | |
| Obturator nerve | Add longus | Adducts leg with knee extended | **L2, L3**, L4 |
| | Add magnus | | |
| Femoral nerve | Iliopsoas | Flexion of hip | **L1, L2**, L3 |
| | Quadriceps | Extends knee | L2, **L3, L4** |
| Superior gluteal nerve | Gluteus medius and minimus | Internal rotation of hip, abduction of hip with knee extended | **L4, L5**, S1 |
| Inferior gluteal nerve | Gluteus maximus | Extension of hip | **L5, S1**, S2 |
| Sciatic nerve proximal to knee | "Hamstrings" | Flexion of knee | L5, **S1**, S2 |
| Tibial nerve (branches off sciatic nerve just above knee) | Gastrocnemius | Plantar flexion | S1, S2 |
| | Soleus | Plantar flexion | S1, S2 |
| | Tibialis posterior | Foot inversion | L4, L5 |
| | Toe flexors | Flexion of toes | L5, **S1, S2** |
| Deep peroneal nerve (distal br of sciatic nerve) | Tibialis anterior | Dorsiflexion | **L4**, L5 |
| | Ext hallucis l | Flexion of big toe | **L5**, S1 |
| | Ext digitorum br | Flexion of toes | L5, S1 |
| Superficial peroneal nerve (distal br of sciatic nerve) | Peroneus l and br | Foot eversion | L5, S1 |

Ext, extensor; Fl, flexor; br, brevis; l, longus; DIP, distal interphalangeal.

[a]Nerve root in bold type usually is dominant.

[b]With arm midway between supination and pronation.

[c]With arm in supination.

## Symmetry vs. Asymmetry

- Polyneuropathies usually are symmetrical, although minor degrees of asymmetry can be encountered.
- Plexopathies usually are unilateral, such that symptoms affect only one extremity.
- Mononeuropathies and multiple mononeuropathies are "patchy" and therefore not symmetrical.
- Radiculopathies most commonly are unilateral.

## Pain

- Pain can be encountered with injury to peripheral nerves, especially sensory neuropathies, radiculopathies, and entrapment mononeuropathies. Plexopathies may or may not be painful; those that are painful usually are due to tumor invasion or compression rather than radiotherapy.
- In general, tumor invasion causes more severe pain than compression. Compression of nerves tends to cause dull aching pain without lancinating pain.
- Pain is much less common with central CNS (central nervous system) processes but can occur.
- Dorsal root ganglion lesions commonly are associated with pain.

## Type of Weakness

- Lower motor neuron (LMN) weakness is due to pathology of peripheral nerves or the motor neuron within the anterior horn of the spinal cord:
  - LMN weakness is associated with atrophy, fasciculations, decreased reflexes, and decreased muscle tone.
  - Pattern: distal weakness is more prominent than proximal weakness. Some demyelinating neuropathies are worse proximally.
  - Clinical tip: patients with polyneuropathies have more difficulty walking on their heels than their toes.
- Upper motor neuron (UMN) weakness is due to pathology at the spinal level or higher:
  - UMN weakness is associated with spasticity, increased reflexes, and Babinski signs. Atrophy may occur as a late sign but usually is less severe than with LMN disease.
  - Pattern: antigravity muscles are affected predominantly—flexors of the arms and extensors of the legs.
  - Facial weakness may be present.
  - Clinical tip: patients may have more difficulty walking on their toes than on their heels.

- Weakness due to myopathy:
  - Weakness is worse proximally than distally, causing difficulty rising from a low chair. The patient may be able to walk on heels and toes normally.
  - No associated sensory loss.
- Weakness due to neuromuscular junction (NMJ) pathology (weakness fluctuates with exertion):
  - In myasthenia gravis, the weakness worsens with exertion. In Lambert-Eaton myasthenic syndrome, the weakness may improve with use.
  - No associated sensory loss.

### Type of Sensory Deficit

- Sensory deficits due to peripheral nerve or dorsal root ganglion lesions: stocking-glove pattern, symmetrical and worse distally than proximally.
- Sensory deficits due to lesions at the spinal level or higher.
- Unilateral intracerebral lesions typically cause sensory findings contralateral to the lesion.
- Ascending numbness beginning in the feet and moving up the legs is commonly due to neuropathy but also can be due to spinal cord compression. If so, there usually is associated spine or radicular pain.

## Polyneuropathy

### Clinical Features

- Polyneuropathies (PNs) are *symmetric* (slight asymmetries may be encountered).
- PNs usually progress from *distal to proximal*.
- PNs usually *begin in the legs* and progress to the arms.
- PNs may be predominantly *sensory, motor, or sensorimotor*.
- PNs may include associated *autonomic* signs and symptoms.
- Sensory PNs can affect large fibers, small fibers, or both:
  - Large fiber neuropathy exhibits loss of proprioception.
  - Small fiber neuropathy exhibits loss of pain and temperature sensation.

### Etiology

Table 48-3 lists the differential diagnosis for polyneuropathy categorized by whether the involvement is predominantly sensory or motor and whether autonomic symptoms are present. Chemotherapy toxicity is a common cause of PN in cancer patients. The pattern of sensory and motor dysfunction usually is characteristic for each drug (see Table 48-3). The diagnosis of a hereditary neuropathy is suggested by a positive family history.

**Table 48-3** Differential Diagnosis of Polyneuropathy in Cancer Patients

| Etiology | Sensory (S), Motor (M), or Autonomic (A) | Comments |
|---|---|---|
| **Chemotherapy agents** | | |
| Vinca alkaloids | S progressing to S/M, with or without A | Reflexes lost early<br>Reversible over months to 2 years |
| Cisplatin | S | Large fiber neuropathy<br>Often painful<br>Lhermitte's sign<br>Dose related |
| Suramin | M | Rapid onset<br>Dose related<br>Demyelinating |
| Taxol | S | Large and small fiber neuropathy<br>Subset also develops proximal motor weakness<br>Reversible |
| Etoposide (VP-16) | S | Uncommon, mild, reversible |
| Cytarabine | S/M | Rare |
| Fludarabine | S or M | Rare |
| Procarbazine | S/M | Uncommon side effect, inflammatory |
| Interleukin-2 | S/M | Compressive neuropathy due to tissue edema (late vascular syndrome) |
| Interferon alpha | S or S/M | Subacute (>4 weeks) |
| Cyclosporine | S/M | Reversible, demyelinating<br>Subacute (>4 weeks) |
| **Nutritional** | | |
| Vitamin $B_{12}$ deficiency | S | Optic atrophy<br>Dorsal column signs<br>+/- megaloblastic anemia |
| **Diabetes** | S/M | Painful |
| Radiotherapy | M > S | Follows radiotherapy to spinal cord, motor neuronopathy |
| Hereditary | S/M | Made worse by chemotherapy |
| Autoimmune | Varies | |
| Paraneoplastic | S or M | |
| Sensory neuronopathy (dorsal root ganglionitis) | S | Subacute sensory loss and dysesthetic pain followed by sensory ataxia<br>Typically precedes tumor diagnosis |

*continues*

**Table 48-3**  Differential Diagnosis of Polyneuropathy in Cancer Patients
*continued*

| Etiology | Sensory (S), Motor (M), or Autonomic (A) | Comments |
|---|---|---|
| Subacute motor neuronopathy | M | Subacute bilateral weakness in the legs and upper extremities<br>Painless |
| Autonomic neuropathy | A | Gastrointestinal dysmotility<br>Pupillary abnormalities<br>Neurogenic bladder<br>Postural hypotension |
| **Tumor invasion** | S/M | Rare<br>Leukemia and lymphoma |

Chemotherapy agents that cause peripheral neuropathy should be avoided in patients with hereditary neuropathies because the peripheral neurotoxicity can be devastating and irreversible.

## Radiculopathy

### Clinical Features

Typically, pain is present, centered over the spine or radiates into the dermatome, or both. Other features are as noted in Table 48-1.

### Etiology

- Tumor:
  - Intradural/extramedullary primary spinal tumors (see Chapter 5).
  - Epidural metastasis (see Chapters 5 and 27).
  - Leptomeningeal metastasis (single or multiple radiculopathies, see Chapter 29).
  - Tumor invasion of nerve root (typically leukemia or lymphoma) usually from paravertebral disease.
- Nerve infarct (typically leukemia or lymphoma).
- Herniated disc, either degenerative or related to spinal instability.
- Compression of nerve root by an osteophyte.
- Compression of nerve root by a compression fracture, either metastatic or osteoporotic.
- Herpes zoster reactivation ("shingles"; see Chapter 32). In general, the rash follows the development of radicular neuropathic pain by 24–72 hours. The cranial nerves and thoracic nerves are the most common sites.
- Radiotherapy (uncommon, usually multiple and due to spinal radiation).

## Mononeuropathy

### Clinical Features

Mononeuropathy (MN) is a focal lesion affecting a single peripheral nerve. Multiple mononeuropathies can sometimes be present and warrant neurologic consultation. The more common mononeuropathies include

- *Median nerve at the wrist (carpal tunnel syndrome):* patients typically present with dysesthetic pain in the palmar surface of the hand that usually is worse at night. The pain frequently radiates into the forearm. In advanced cases, weakness and atrophy of the median-innervated muscles (see Table 48-2) in the hand develop. Mild cases can be managed conservatively with nonsteroid anti-inflammatory drugs and wrist splinting. Resistant cases may require decompression.
- *Ulnar nerve at the elbow:* usually due to trauma (acute or chronic) to the elbow. Patients develop weakness and atrophy of all ulnar-innervated muscles (see Table 48-2) with resulting disability of the hand. Sensory loss occurs along the ulnar aspect of the hand below the wrist. If numbness extends above the wrist, a C8-T1 radiculopathy or lower brachial plexopathy should be considered.
- *Ulnar nerve at the wrist:* weakness of the small muscles of the hand without sensory loss.
- *Lateral femoral cutaneous nerve at the inguinal ligament (meralgia paresthetica):* numbness and sensitivity to touch over the anterior-lateral thigh. No motor deficit is present and reflexes are normal.
- *Common peroneal nerve at the head of the tibia:* loss of dorsiflexion and eversion of the foot, numbness on the dorsum of the foot. Pain may be mild to severe.
- *Femoral nerve:* occurs more often in cancer patients than in noncancer patients, usually due to infiltration by tumor, nerve infarction, trauma related to pelvic surgery, or hemotoma secondary to surgery or anticoagulation.
- *Obturator nerve:* pain is referred to the inner thigh and may be the only symptom. When present, weakness involves the hip adductors and, to a lesser degree, the internal and external rotators of the hip.
- *Sciatic nerve:* loss of flexion at the knee, motor loss below the knee, weakness of the gluteal muscles. When the lesion is at the sciatic notch or pelvis, there is pain in the buttock and posterior thigh. When the lesion is below the sciatic notch, the gluteal muscles are not affected.
- *Tibial nerve:* loss of plantar flexion and inversion of the foot and loss of sensation over the plantar aspect of the foot.

## Etiology

- Tumor invasion or compression: typically more neurologic dysfunction with invasion than compression.
- Amyloidosis (multiple myeloma).
- Nerve infarct (leukemia, lymphoma).
- Trauma examples:
  - Carpal tunnel syndrome due to repetitive wrist trauma.
  - Surgical: mastectomy frequently damages the intercostal-brachial nerve causing a tight, burning sensation that is mild to severe.
  - Postoperative pressure palsies: ulnar, radial, femoral, sciatic, peroneal, and obturator.
- Chemotherapy usually does not cause MN unless the agent is infused in direct proximity to a peripheral nerve.
- Compressive neuropathies also can be caused by systemic conditions that result in soft tissue edema, such as hypothyroidism, congestive heart failure, and pregnancy. The vascular leak syndrome associated with interleukin-2 can cause compressive neuropathy by this mechanism.

## Plexopathies

Figures 48-1 and 48-2 provide schematic illustrations of the anatomy of the brachial and lumbar plexuses. Most plexopathies are unilateral, although some are bilateral. Pain may or may not be present, depending on the etiology. Plexopathies can be complete or partial. In cancer patients, the main differential diagnosis is between radiation injury and recurrent tumor.

## Brachial Plexopathy

- Tumor
  - Painful.
  - Tends to involve upper portion of brachial plexus.
  - Progressive.
  - When Horner's syndrome is present, cervical epidural tumor should be suspected.
- Radiotherapy:
  - Acute: acute, painful, reversible brachial plexus palsy that begins during radiotherapy for Hodgkin's disease occurs occasionally.
  - Early-delayed: reversible plexopathy due to radiation may occur 4–6 months following radiotherapy to the involved plexus. Paresthesias and sometimes pain are present, and weakness is mild to moderate. Treatment is symptomatic.

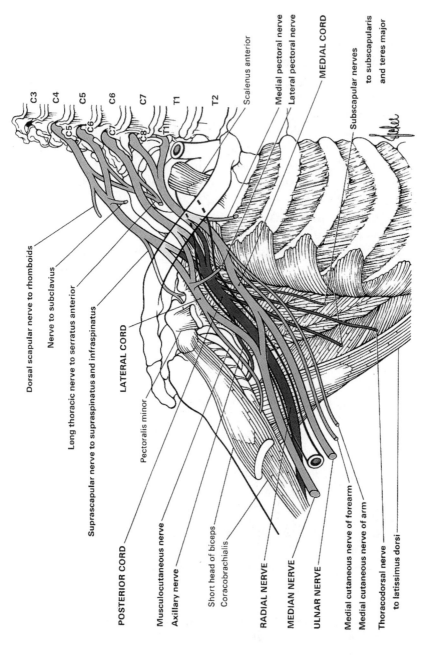

**Figure 48-1** Schematic illustration of the anatomy of the brachial plexus. (Reprinted with permission from the Guarantors of Brain. *Aids to the Examination of the Peripheral Nervous System.* Philadelphia: W.B. Saunders, 1987:4.)

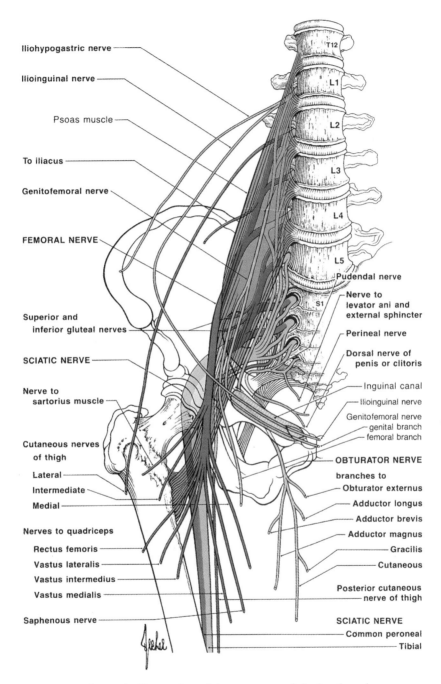

**Figure 48-2**  Schematic illustration of the anatomy of the lumbar plexus. (Reprinted with permission from the Guarantors of Brain. *Aids to the Examination of the Peripheral Nervous System.* Philadelphia: W.B. Saunders, 1987:31.)

- Late-delayed: irreversible plexopathy may occur within months to years following radiotherapy, associated with paresthesias but rarely pain. The entire extremity may become paralyzed. Pain is dull and aching or neuropathic.
- Surgical and trauma examples:
  - Brachial plexus palsy following prolonged positioning for thoracotomy or mastectomy.
  - Compressive brachial plexopathy due to hematoma formation following attempted subclavian catheter placement can occur rarely. This condition usually reverses within a few weeks and treatment is symptomatic.
  - Transient brachial plexopathy due to lidocaine injection for internal jugular vein catheter placement usually lasts only a few hours.
- Brachial neuritis (idiopathic).
- Brachial after interferon alpha.
- Lymphedema also can cause arm pain but is not associated with neurologic deficit.

### Lumbosacral Plexopathy

Lumbosacral plexopathies typically cause unilateral muscle weakness, sensory changes, and reflex attenuation. These signs and symptoms are not confined to the distribution of a single nerve root or peripheral nerve.

- Tumor, almost always painful: direct infiltration, compression.
- Trauma or surgery: damage during surgical procedures of the abdomen and pelvis.
- Radiotherapy: early-delayed or late-delayed as described previously. Weakness usually is more prominent than pain and usually is bilateral (as compared with tumor involvement, which usually is unilateral).
- Vascular: compression by abdominal aortic aneurysm. Pain radiates into the anterior thigh and hip, mild weakness of hip flexion, and decreased sensation over the anterior thigh.
- Idiopathic.

### Evaluation

Laboratory investigations are guided by the suspected etiology but all patients should be tested for treatable neuropathies: $B_{12}$ level, complete blood count, thyroid function tests, and blood glucose or hemoglobin A1C. An electromyogram (EMG) is helpful in confirming the presence of peripheral nerve pathology, distinguishing axonal from demyelinating neuropathies, and quantifying the extent of sensory and motor nerve pathology. All plexopathies should be evaluated with imaging. Magnetic resonance imaging (MRI) is best and can identify tumor or radiation-related fibrosis. Hematoma is best seen on computed tomography (CT) scan.

## Treatment

Therapy for peripheral nerve dysfunction depends on the diagnosis. Consultation with a neurologist for diagnosis and management is recommended. Tumors involving the brachial plexus often are treated with radiotherapy. When nerve injury is due to chemotherapeutic agents, stopping the exposure usually reverses the condition, although full recovery may take 1–2 years. All patients with significant peripheral dysfunction should undergo physical therapy; bracing may be required for motor impairment. Pharmacologic approaches to neuropathic pain are covered in Chapter 54.

## Suggested Reading

Amato AA, Collins MP. Neuropathies associated with malignancy. *Semin Neurol.* 1998;18(1):125–144.

Freilich RJ, Balmaceda C, Seidman AD, et al. Motor neuropathy due to docetaxel and paclitaxel. *Neurology.* 1996;47(1):115–118.

Guarantors of Brain. *Aids to the Examination of the Peripheral Nervous System.* Philadelphia: W.B. Saunders, 1987.

Posner JB. *Neurologic Complications of Cancer.* Philadelphia: F.A. Davis, 1995.

# 49

## Seizures and
## Other Spells

Many brain tumor patients experience a seizure during their illness; and some brain tumors, such as oligodendrogliomas, are more epileptogenic than others. Overall, 10–20% of brain tumor patients present with seizures and another 10–20% experience a seizure during the course of their illness. The complications of seizures are more significant for patients with brain tumors. In particular, the postictal state can last over 24 hours and occasionally is associated with a permanent increase in neurologic deficit. Recurrent seizures also can raise intracranial pressure and cause clinical decompensation. Other spells of neurologic dysfunction must be distinguished from seizures.

### Diagnosis

- A correct diagnosis of seizure depends on an accurate history. Details of the event are best obtained from an observer who has witnessed one or more of the patient's spells. The patient often can provide the history if the episode did not cause loss of consciousness. However, patients with complex partial seizures may be amnestic for some or all of the episode.
- Episodes of transient neurologic dysfunction in brain tumor patients should be treated as seizures, unless an alternative diagnosis is unequivocal.
- Electroencephalogram (EEG) can be helpful in certain circumstances. However, a normal or nonepileptiform EEG pattern does not exclude seizures.

## Types of Seizures

Table 49-1 provides a practical approach to categorizing seizure type. Refer to "Proposal for Revised Classification of Epilepsies and Epileptic Syndromes" (Commission, 1989) for a more detailed classification. Seizures are classified as partial or generalized. In general, seizures related to a brain tumor are partial in onset but secondary generalization is common:

- *Partial* implies seizure onset from a specific location in the brain:
  - Partial seizures are further categorized by whether or not consciousness is impaired (see Table 49-1).

**Table 49-1**   Types of Seizures

| *Seizure* | | |
|---|---|---|
| **Partial seizures:** | | |
| Simple partial seizures (consciousness not impaired) | With motor symptoms<br>With somatosensory or special sensory symptoms<br>With autonomic symptoms<br>With psychic symptoms | |
| Complex partial seizures (consciousness impaired) | Begin as simple partial seizures and progress to impairment of consciousness | With no other features<br>With features as in simple partial seizures<br>With automatisms[a] |
| | With impairment of consciousness at onset | With no other features<br>With features as in simple partial seizures<br>With automatisms |
| | Partial seizures with secondary generalization | |
| **Generalized seizures (convulsive or nonconvulsive):** | | |
| Absence seizures[b] | | Typical absence seizures<br>Atypical absence seizures |
| Myoclonic seizures[b] | | |
| Clonic seizures | | |
| Tonic seizures | | |
| Tonic-clonic seizures | | |
| Atonic seizures[b] | | |

[a]Motor behaviors that are repetitive, nonreflexive, and nonvolitional.

[b]Rare in brain tumor patients.

**Table 49-2**     Differential Diagnosis of Episodic Neurologic Dysfunction in
Cancer Patients

| |
|---|
| Seizures |
| Episodic increases in intracranial pressure, plateau waves |
| Syncope: cardiac arrhythmia, hypotensive or hypovolemic, orthostatic hypotension, vasovagal |
| Vascular: transient ischemic attacks |
| Migraine |
| Hypoglycemia |
| Vertigo |
| Hyperventilation, anxiety, panic attacks |
| Movement disorders: myoclonus, asterixis, hemiballismus (rare) |
| Pseudoseizures |

- – Partial seizures can terminate or undergo secondary generalization.
- *Generalized* implies involvement of both cerebral hemispheres at on-set; consciousness is impaired at seizure onset:
  - – Patients may not experience premonitory symptoms before a generalized seizure.
  - – New onset of absence seizures in adulthood is rare; consider complex partial seizures instead.

### Differential Diagnosis of Episodic Neurologic Dysfunction

- Table 49-2 provides a differential diagnosis of episodic neurologic dysfunction.
- These conditions are less common than seizures, particularly when the patient has a known primary or metastatic brain tumor.
- Pseudoseizures are rare in patients with brain tumors.
- Episodes of knee buckling ("my legs give out on me") without loss of consciousness are generally not epileptic and may be due to episodic increases in intracranial pressure, early spinal cord compression, or proximal myopathy due to corticosteroids.

## Causes of Seizures in Cancer Patients

One or more of the following contributory factors may be present in a given patient:

- Tumor
  - Progression of known intracranial malignancy.
  - New brain, dural, or leptomeningeal metastasis.
  - Tumor embolus.
- Metabolic:
  - Hyponatremia (may be caused by carbamazepine).
  - Hypoxia.
  - Hypocalcemia.
  - Hypomagnesemia.
  - Uremia.
  - Hyperglycemia or hypoglycemia.
- Vascular (see Chapter 50):
  - Stroke.
  - Intracranial hemorrhage.
  - Intratumoral hemorrhage.
  - Venous sinus or cerebral vein thrombosis.
- Central nervous system infections (see Chapter 32).
  - Bacterial, viral, fungal, parasitic.
- Chemotherapy agents:
  - Methotrexate.
  - Cytarabine.
  - L-asparaginase.
  - Taxol.
  - Ifosphamide.
  - Nitrosoureas.
  - Cisplatin.
- Radiation effects: radiation necrosis or encephalopathy.
- Other drugs:
  - Tricyclic antidepressants.
  - Antibiotics: penicillins, imipenem-cilastatin.
  - Antipsychotics.
  - Opioids.
  - Butyrophenones.
  - Phenothiazines.
  - Meperidine.
- Low anticonvulsant levels:
  - Serum levels of some anticonvulsants lowered by dexamethasone.
  - Some chemotherapeutic agents lower anticonvulsant levels.
  - Patient noncompliance or misunderstanding of instructions.
  - Inability to take oral medications due to nausea or dysphagia.

## Laboratory Tests

- Electrolytes, calcium.
- Glucose.
- BUN and creatinine.
- Liver function tests.
- Anticonvulsant drug levels.

## Treatment of Seizures

Patients who have experienced more than one seizure are started on anticonvulsant agents. Anticonvulsant dosing, therapeutic levels, side effects, and drug interactions are summarized in Table 49-3. The goal of anticonvulsant therapy is to achieve acceptable seizure control with minimal side effects.

- Patients with correctable causes of seizures (e.g., hyponatremia), normal neurologic examination, *and* no structural abnormalities on neuroimaging exams do not require long-term anticonvulsant therapy. If short-term therapy is selected for those patients that have reversible causes, the following guidelines apply:
  - Phenytoin generally is used for such patients.
  - Phenytoin is *ineffective* in the management of seizures due to alcohol withdrawal or drug toxicity such as theophylline and isoniazide.
  - Anticonvulsant therapy is tapered off and withdrawn following a short observation period.
- Patients with structural lesions, such as primary or metastatic brain tumors, require long-term anticonvulsant treatment because the risk of seizure recurrence is high:
  - Phenytoin, phenobarbital, and carbamazepine commonly used.
  - Levataracitam, a newer agent, has fewer drug interactions.
  - Carbamazepine or valproic acid is preferred for patients with seizures of temporal lobe origin.
  - Monotherapy is preferred over polytherapy. The agent initially chosen should be used at the maximum dose that the patient can tolerate before adding another drug or changing to another agent.
  - Some patients have refractory seizures and require polytherapy.
- Many patients experience cognitive dysfunction on anticonvulsant medications.

**Table 49-3** Summary of Selected Anticonvulsant Agents

| Agent | Initiation of Treatment[a] | Starting Dose Maintenance Dose Range[b] | Therapeutic Reference Range (mg/ml)[c] | Common/Important Side Effects and Comments |
|---|---|---|---|---|
| Phenytoin | Emergency: 15–20 mg/kg IV at < 50 mg/min. Oral loading: 300 mg PO × 3 doses over 8–10 hrs | Start: 5 mg/kg. Range: 200–700/d | 10–20 | Sedation, ataxia, drug interactions. Allergic rash (20%) |
| Phenobarbital | Emergency: 20 mg/kg at < 100 mg/min, anticipate acute sedation and respiratory depression | Start: 60 mg/d. Range: 60–240/d | 15–40 | Adults—sedation. Children—hyperactivity and agression or sedation. Allergic rash (20%) |
| Carbamazepine | Cannot be loaded orally due to GI intolerance | Start: 100–200 bid. Increase dose by 100–200 mg qd until goal dose reached. Range: 400–1500, divided bid to tid | Single agent: 8–12. Polytherapy: 6–8 | Diplopia, dizziness, ataxia, GI upset, hyponatremia. Allergic rash (20%) |
| Oxcarbazepine | Cannot be effectively loaded orally | 300 bid, increase to 600 bid | — | Similar to carbamazepine. 30% cross sensitivity to carbamazepine |
| Valproic acid | Cannot be effectively loaded orally due to GI intolerance | Start: 250 mg bid to tid. Range: 500–3000 divided tid | 50–140 | GI upset, tremor, weight gain, thrombocytopenia, hair thinning |
| | IV form: emergency, 10 mg/kg up to 20 mg/kg | 5 mg/kg/d divided tid or switch to oral form | 50–140 | As for oral |

*continues*

**Table 49-3**   Summary of Selected Anticonvulsant Agents   *continued*

| Agent | Initiation of Treatment[a] | Starting Dose Maintenance Dose Range[b] | Therapeutic Reference Range (mg/ml)[c] | Common/Important Side Effects and Comments |
|---|---|---|---|---|
| Gabapentin | Not applicable (oral) | 100 mg PO tid Increase by 100 mg/d every 3 days to reach goal dose Range: 900–1800/d | Not applicable[d] | Somnolence, fatigue, ataxia, dizziness, GI upset Also helpful for neuropathic pain |
| Topirimate | Not applicable (oral) | 25 mg bid, increase by 25 mg/dose every 2–3 days to maximum dose of 200 mg bid | Not applicable | Cognitive slowing, tremor, distal paresthesias, risk of renal calculi |
| Levetiracetam | Not applicable (oral) | 250 mg (½ pill) bid and increase by ½ pill increments to maximum of 1000 mg bid | Not applicable | Sedation, dizziness |
| Lamotrigine | Not applicable (oral) | Start: 25–50 mg/d[e] Increase by 50 mg/d every 1–2 weeks Range: 200–700 mg/d | Not applicable | Tremor, dizziness, ataxia, diplopia, headache, GI upset Rash (20%)[f] Stevens-Johnson syndrome (rare) |

GI, gastrointestinal.

[a]Only phenytoin, phenobarbital, benzodiazepines, and valproic acid are reliably effective IV treatment for status epilepticus or frequent seizures that need urgent control. See Table 49-4 for status epilepticus.

[b]Once daily dosing at bedtime is used for phenytoin and phenobarbital. Dividing doses may help seizure control in some patients but may contribute to daytime sedation. Carbamezapine is given bid to tid and valproic acid is given tid to qid.

[c]Therapeutic levels are used as references. The therapeutic level for an individual patient is that which results in seizure control with acceptable side effects.

[d]Drug levels not readily available or not useful.

[e]When used with valproic acid, start at 25 mg/d every other day and increase by 25 mg/d every 1–2 weeks to a total dose of 100–150 mg/d.

[f]Rash may abate with observation, rarely proceeds to Stevens-Johnson syndrome.

## Prophylactic Anticonvulsant Therapy

- All the available anticonvulsant agents can cause serious side effects. In randomized prospective studies, prophylactic anticonvulsants failed to provide benefit for patients with primary or metastatic brain tumors, and they therefore should be avoided. However, prophylactic anticonvulsants are useful in the perioperative period after craniotomy, since postoperative seizures can cause increased intracranial pressure (ICP) and neurologic deterioration. They can be tapered off 2–3 weeks after surgery.
- Patients with hemorrhagic tumors and metastases from melanoma are at a high risk for seizures, and prophylactic anticonvulsant therapy should be considered on an individualized basis.
- Oligodendrogliomas are highly epileptogenic tumors. Episodic neurologic symptoms should be regarded with suspicion and treated as seizures.
- Certain situations pose an increased risk of seizures in patients with intracranial tumors, including acute increased ICP, general anesthesia, and during radiotherapy (particularly prior to single-fraction stereotactic radiation).

## Status Epilepticus

The initial approach to status epilepticus (SE) is summarized in Table 49-4.

- SE is a neurologic emergency. Patients should be hospitalized and placed in the intensive care unit for treatment. Although the mortality rate for SE has declined over the past three decades, the mortality remains higher for patients with structural lesions, such as brain tumors.
- Nonconvulsive SE may present as confusion or may mimic psychiatric illness and requires continuous EEG monitoring for diagnosis and management.

**Table 49-4**   Initial Treatment of Status Epilepticus

1. Maintain ABCs: airway, breathing and circulation. Assess vital signs. Institute treatment to protect airway, ventilation, and maintain blood pressure as appropriate.

2. Insert an intravenous catheter, obtain STAT labs (electrolytes, BUN/creatinine, glucose, anticonvulsant drug levels). Test arterial blood gases.

3. Verify the diagnosis of SE. Observe at least one seizure.

4. Infuse thiamine 100 mg IV and dextrose (50 cc of D50W).

5. Obtain a history, if possible. Does the patient have known epilepsy? Is the patient on anticonvulsant medication? Does the patient have a known intracranial lesion? Are there known allergies?

6. Begin anticonvulsant therapy: Lorazepam 0.1 mg/kg at 2 mg/minute.

7. Begin antibiotics if bacterial meningitis is suspected.

8. If seizures persist, begin phenytoin 20 mg/kg at 50 mg/minute. Monitor for hypotension. If alcohol or other drug withdrawal or toxicity is suspected, do not give phenytoin and proceed with step 9. If seizures have stopped with lorazepam, phenytoin also should be started in any patient not on anticonvulsant agents or thought to have been noncompliant with anticonvulsant therapy.

9. If seizures persist, intubate the patient (if not already done) and begin ventilation.

10. If seizures persist, begin phenobarbital 20 mg/kg at 100 mg/minute. Monitor for hypotension.

11. Following phenobarbital,
    - If seizures persist, institute continuous EEG monitoring and prepare to induce pharmacologic coma (pentobarbital, propofol, midazolam). Specialty care from a physician experienced in the management of refractory SE is needed at this point.
    - If clinical seizures stop, obtain an EEG to exclude ongoing electrographic seizure activity.
    - Evaluate for etiology of SE. Obtain neuro-imaging study as soon as the patient is stable and perform lumbar puncture if appropriate.
    - Monitor anticonvulsant levels closely.

# Reference

Commission on Classification and Terminology of the International League Against Epilepsy. Proposal for revised classification of epilepsies and epileptic syndromes. *Epilepsia.* 1989;30(4):389.

## Suggested Reading

Anderson GD. A mechanistic approach to antiepileptic drug interactions. *Ann Pharmacotherapy.* 1998;32:554–563.

Brodie MJ, Dichter MA. Antiepileptic drugs. *N Engl J Med.* 1996; 334(3);168–175.

Chalifoux R, Elisevich K. Effect of ionizing radiation on partial seizures attributable to malignant cerebral tumors. *Stereotact Funct Neurosurg.* 1996–1997;67(3–4):169–182.

Chokroverty S. *Management of Epilepsy.* Boston: Butterworth–Heinemann, 1996.

Delgado-Escueta AV, Fong CY. Status epilepticus: recent trends and prospects. *Neurologia.* 1997;12(Suppl 6):62–73.

Dichter MA, Brodie MJ. New antiepileptic drugs. *N Engl J Med.* 1996;334(24): 1583–1590.

Glantz MJ, Cole BF, Friedberg MH, et al. A randomized, blinded, placebo-controlled trial of divalproex sodium prophylaxis in adults with newly diagnosed brain tumors. *Neurology.* 1996;46(4):985–991.

Jagoda A, Richardson L. The evaluation and treatment of seizures in the emergency department. *Mt Sinai J Med.* 1997;64(4–5):249–257.

Kaplan PW. Nonconvulsive status epilepticus. *Semin Neurol.* 1996;16(1):33–40.

Natsch S, Yechiel AH, Keyser A, et al. Newer anticonvulsant drugs. Role of pharmacology, drug interactions and adverse reactions in drug choice. *Drug Safety.* 1997;17(4):228–240.

Riva R, Albani F, Contin M, et al. Pharmacokinetic interactions between antiepileptic drugs. Clinical considerations. *Clin Pharmacokinet.* 1996;31(6): 470–493.

Tasker RC. Emergency treatment of acute seizures and status epilepticus. *Arch Dis Child.* 1998;79(1):78–83.

Walker MC. The epidemiology and management of status epilepticus. *Curr Opin Neurol.* 1998;11(2):149–154.

# 50

# Stroke and Other Cerebrovascular Complications

Symptomatic strokes and other cerebrovascular events occur in 7–10% of cancer patients. Although the spectrum of pathology differs from that of patients with no cancer, the most common cause of stroke in cancer patients is atherosclerosis. Recognition of a cerebrovascular event directs appropriate evaluation and management and avoids treatment for an erroneous diagnosis. Perhaps the most important example of this is distinguishing a hemorrhagic infarct from a hemorrhagic brain metastasis. Such a distinction avoids radiotherapy for nonmalignant disease. Specific treatments and preventative measures are indicated for some types of strokes.

## Overview

Table 50-1 and Figure 50-1 summarize the more common cerebrovascular syndromes that affect cancer patients. Patients with typical thrombotic or embolic infarctions experience the acute onset of neurologic symptoms referable to a single vascular territory. Pain or headache usually is minimal. Signs and symptoms of increased intracranial pressure (ICP) are not present initially but may develop over the first 24 hours in large strokes. The extent of neurologic deficit is greatest at the onset and usually improves with time. This is an important distinguishing feature from metastasis, in which signs and symptoms are progressive and subacute in onset. The most common stroke syndrome involves the territory of the middle cerebral artery, resulting in a hemiparesis that involves the arm and face more than the leg,

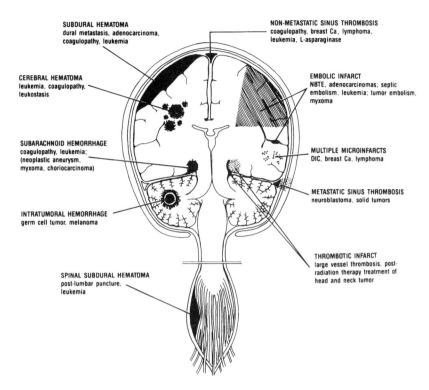

**Figure 50-1** Cerebrovascular disorders encountered in patients with cancer. The left side of the figure illustrates hemorrhagic lesions and the right portion illustrates ischemic lesions. (Reprinted with permission from Posner JB. *Neurologic Complications of Cancer.* Philadelphia: F.A. Davis, 1995:200.)

hemisensory loss, and aphasia (dominant hemisphere) or apraxia (nondominant hemisphere). Adams, Victor, and Ropper present a detailed discussion of stroke syndromes and the related vascular anatomy.

## Approach to the Patient

When a cerebrovascular event is suspected in a cancer patient, hospitalization usually is warranted for diagnosis and management.

### History

- Nature of onset: abrupt vs. gradual.
- Presence of headache.
- Recent treatments, medications, fever, infections, history of anticoagulation, falls, previous stroke, cardiac disease, hypertension, diabetes.

**Table 50-1**   Cerebrovascular Events in Cancer Patients

| Mechanism | Associated Tumors | Associated Conditions |
|---|---|---|
| **Embolic infarction**[a] | | |
| Tumor embolus | Lung cancer or pulmonary metastasis<br>Right atrial myxoma | |
| Septic embolus | Most common in leukemia | Subacute bacterial endocarditis<br>Fungal vasculitis of cerebral vessels |
| Nonbacterial thrombotic endocarditis | Any tumor, usually solid tumors | Other end organ emboli may be present |
| Embolic stroke | Not tumor related | Patent foramen ovale<br>Left ventricular dysfunction<br>Atrial fibrillation<br>Valvular heart disease<br>Carotid and aortic arch disease |
| **Thrombotic-arterial lesion** | | |
| Disseminated intravascular coagulation | Any tumor, most common in lymphoma and breast cancer | Sepsis<br>NBTE |
| Systemic chemotherapy | Any tumor | Cisplatin<br>Bleomycin<br>Mitomycin |
| Intra-arterial chemotherapy | Primary and metastatic brain tumors | Cisplatin<br>Carboplatin<br>Carmastine<br>Methotrexate |
| Atherosclerosis | Most common cause of stroke; not related to tumor type | Smoking<br>Diabetes<br>Hypertension<br>Radiotherapy to head and neck can accelerate atherosclerosis |
| Small vessel occlusive disease (lacunar infarction) | | Diabetes<br>Hypertension |
| **Thrombotic-venous lesion** | | |
| Venous sinus or cerebral vein thrombosis[b] | Dural metastasis<br>Hyperviscosity states: myeloma, lymphoma | Hypercoagulable states due to chemotherapy (L-asparaginase)<br>Non-tumor-related hypercoagulable states |

*continues*

**Table 50-1** Cerebrovascular Events in Cancer Patients *continued*

| Mechanism | Associated Tumors | Associated Conditions |
|---|---|---|
| **Hemorrhagic lesions** | | |
| Intratumoral hemorrhage | Primary and meta-static tumors[c] | Increased risk with coagulop-athy and thrombocytopenia |
| Leukostasis | Leukemia, especially AML | WBC usually >100/µl |
| Thrombocytopenia (spontaneous cerebral hemorrhage) | Myelosuppression from bone marrow infiltration by tumor, most commonly leukemia, lymphoma | Myelosuppression from chemo-therapy, radiotherapy (risk relates to the degree of thrombocytopenia) |
| Hypertensive hemorrhage | | Hypertension |
| Subdural hematoma | Dural metastases: prostate, breast cancer | Coagulopathy Falls or trauma |

NBTE, nonbacterial thrombotic endocarditis; AML, acute myelogenous leukemia; WBC, white blood cell.

[a]Both embolic and thrombotic infarctions can develop into hemorrhagic lesions.

[b]May cause a venous hemorrhagic infarction.

[c]Tumors that tend to hemorrhage include melanoma, thyroid, choriocarcinoma, lung cancer, and some primary brain tumors.

## Examination

- General exam
  - Signs of other emboli (eye grounds, nailbeds).
  - Cardiac examination: murmur, cardiomegaly.
  - Auscultation for carotid bruits.
  - Funduscopic examination: hemorrhages, papilledema, arterial emboli or narrowing.
  - Evaluation for potential source of sepsis.
  - Evaluation for peripheral venous thrombosis or catheter related clots.
- Detailed neurologic examination.

## Laboratory Tests

- Complete blood count including platelet count.
- Coagulation studies: protime and prothrombin time (international normalized ratio for patients anticoagulated with warfarin), disseminated intravascular coagulation (DIC) evaluation (D-dimer).

- Urinalysis: hematuria suggests concomitant emboli to the kidneys, as occurs in subacute bacterial endocarditis (SBE) or nonbacterial thrombotic endocarditis (NBTE).
- Erythrocyte sedimentation rate if vasculitis or SBE is suspected.
- Echocardiogram to look for source of embolus (SBE, NBTE). Consider transesophageal echocardiogram (TEE), especially for NBTE.
- Carotid doppler examinations to exclude critical stenosis.
- Computed tomography (CT) or magnetic resonance imaging (MRI) scans of the brain should be performed as soon as possible. Magnetic resonance angiography may be appropriate.

### Initial Management

- Therapeutic anticoagulation should be stopped pending initial evaluation if a hemorrhagic event is suspected.
- Close observation for neurologic deterioration.
- Careful monitoring of fluid status.
- Neurologic consultation.

## Suggested Reading

Adams RD, Victor M, Ropper AH. *Principles of Neurology* (6th ed). New York: McGraw-Hill, 1997.

Chaturvedi S, Ansell J, Recht L. Should cerebral ischemic events in cancer patients be considered a manifestation of hypercoagulability? *Stroke.* 1994; 25(6):1215–1218.

# 51

# Urinary Problems

Urinary symptoms are common problems in neuro-oncology patients. They may be the initial symptoms of neurologic disease, provide diagnostic clues, and are of significant concern to the patient. Urinary symptoms usually are not volunteered by the patient because they are not recognized as "neurologic"; direct questioning is required. This chapter focuses on the practical aspects of diagnosing and managing urinary problems in neuro-oncology patients. Consultation with a urologist experienced in neurologic urology may be helpful. Complicated patients and those who do not respond to initial interventions may require urologic evaluation to maintain continence and preserve renal function.

## Evaluation

### History

Questions to ask:

- Do you have problems controlling your urine? Controlling your bladder?
- When you urinate, does your bladder still feel full?
- Is there hesitancy in starting the stream or dribbling after you are done?
- Do you have trouble getting to the bathroom in time?
- Do you feel an urge to urinate and then have trouble urinating?
- Do you leak urine when you cough or sneeze?
- How often do you urinate?
- How many times do you get up at night to urinate?
- When you urinate, does it seem like a lot or a little?
- Do you have pain or burning with urination? How long does it last?
- Is your urine cloudy or bloody?
- What medications are you taking?

## Examination

- Neurologic examination for myelopathy or intracranial process.
- Urinary retention and back pain in a cancer patient raises suspicion of cord compression.
- Evaluate causes of impaired mobility.
- Check for bladder distension.
- Check for fecal impaction.
- In women, check vaginal mucosa for atrophy and bladder prolapse.
- In men, examine for prostate hypertrophy.

## Laboratory Tests

- Urinalysis to exclude infection.
- Blood glucose to exclude diabetes mellitus.
- Serum sodium to exclude diabetes insipidus.
- Measure postvoid residual.
- Cystoscopy to evaluate hematuria or incontinence that does not respond to medications.
- Spine or brain magnetic resonance imaging (MRI) scans to evaluate for suspected spinal cord compression or intracranial lesion, as indicated by the clinical situation.

## Management

### Goals

- Maintain continence, comfort, and patient dignity.
- Preserve normal renal function.
- Limit autonomic dysreflexia.
- Limit symptomatic infections.

### Simple Measures

- Treat infection, if present.
- Manage diabetes mellitus or diabetes insipidus, if present.
- Timed voidings: having patients void every 2–3 hours is effective management for patients with mobility problems and may also help patients with overflow incontinence.
- Make toilet facilities convenient for the patient by using a bedside commode, urinal, or bedpan. In bedridden patients, consider condom catheters (intermittent, if possible) or indwelling catheters.

- In patients with urinary retention, try stimulation (Credé's method, Valsalva's maneuver, tapping the bladder) or clean intermittent catheterization.
- Use absorbent pads for small-volume incontinence such as stress incontinence and adult diapers for larger volume incontinence.
- Treat and prevent constipation.

## Review Medications

- Stop or reduce anticholingergic medications in patients with overflow incontinence.
- Narcotics also may cause urinary retention, but most patients habituate to this or respond to timed voiding.
- Avoid diuretics or schedule dosing early in the day and at times the patient will be close to the bathroom.

## Pharmacological and Surgical Management

- Manipulate detrusor function (outlet resistance):
  - Bethanechol (urecholine) 10 mg PO tid (up to 50 mg PO tid) for overflow incontinence.
  - Oxybutynin (Ditropan) 2.5–5 mg PO tid to qid for urge incontinence.
  - Imiprimine 10–20 mg PO qhs for neurogenic bladder or stress incontinence.
  - Artificial sphincters.
  - Periuretheral collagen injection.
- For dysuria,
  - Treat infection.
  - Atrophic vaginitis: ethinyl estradiol 0.02 mg PO qd or conjugated estrogen 0.625 mg PO qd. An estrase ring can be used in breast cancer patients if oral estrogens are contraindicated.
  - Phenazopyridine (Pyridium) 100–200 mg PO qid (turns the urine red-orange).
- For bladder spasms,
  - Treat infection and constipation.
  - Remove indwelling catheter or partially deflate balloon.
  - Imiprimine 10–20 mg PO qhs.
  - Amitriptyline 10–25 mg PO qhs.
  - Oxybutynin 2.5–5.0 mg PO tid.
  - Hyoscyamin (Levsin) 0.125–0.25 mg PO tid to qid.

## Suggested Reading

Stamm WE, Hooton TM. Management of urinary tract infections in adults. *New Eng J Med.* 1993;329(18)1328–1334.

Wein AJ. Lower urinary tract function and pharmacologic management of lower urinary tract dysfunction. *Urol Clin North Am.* 1987;14(2):273–296.

# 52

# Visual Symptoms

Visual problems are common in neuro-oncology patients and can arise at multiple locations along the visual pathway. They may be indicative of specific neurologic or ophthalmologic dysfunction. Diagnosis of visual symptoms may disclose previously undiagnosed pathology within the central nervous system (CNS) and appropriate management significantly enhances the patient's quality of life. Consultation with an ophthalmologist or neuro-ophthalmologist sometimes is necessary.

## General Approach

### History

Patients should be questioned regarding the nature of their visual symptoms, onset and duration, and whether they have associated facial pain or numbness. Determining whether the problem is in one or both eyes or a problem with extraocular motility sometimes is possible based on the history.

## Examination

Important steps in the assessment of visual symptoms include

1. Visual acuity: Snellen's chart at 20 feet or a handheld "near" card. Test each eye separately, using the patient's reading glasses if necessary.
2. Visual field exam (bedside):
   - Test each eye separately and ask patient to count fingers in all four quadrants.
   - Testing with both eyes open can identify visual neglect.
   - Record visual fields as shown in Figure 52-1.

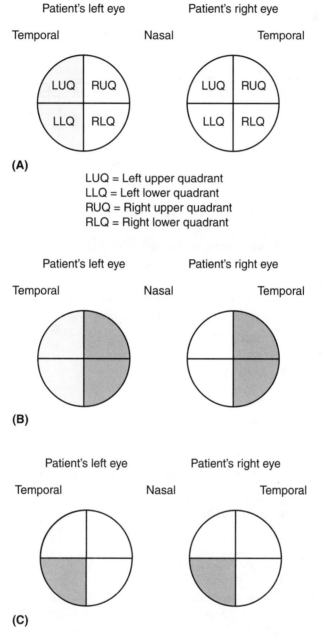

**Figure 52-1**   Recording of visual field deficits: **A**, quadrants of the visual field; **B**, example of a right homonymous hemianopsia; **C**, example of a left lower quadrantanopsia.

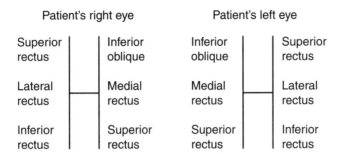

**Figures 52-2**   Cardinal positions of gaze and extraocular muscles (drawn from the perspective of the examiner facing the patient).

3. Extraocular movements:
   - Test each eye separately. The patient covers one eye and follows the examiner's finger in a letter *H* (see Figure 52-2).
     The third nerve supplies inferior oblique, superior rectus, inferior rectus, medial rectus, and the levator of the eyelid.
     The sixth nerve supplies the lateral rectus.
     The fourth nerve supplies the superior oblique.
4. Pupil exam:
   - Note pupil size and shape in light and dark and reaction to light (direct and consensual).
   - Examine for a relative afferent pupillary defect (RAPD or Marcus Gunn pupil: the affected pupil does not react to direct light but does react to consensual light).
   - Check the near reflex (pupils constrict with convergence).
5. Funduscopic exam for papilledema, venous pulsations, retinopathy, cotton-wool spots.

Steps 4 and 5 should be done last to avoid the effect of bright light on the visual acuity and visual field exams.

## Loss of Visual Acuity

- If the problem is in one eye, the lesion is anterior to the optic chiasm.
- Bilateral visual loss is likely due to a lesion in the chiasm or postchiasmal optic tract but can be due to pathology involving both retinas.
- Ischemic or inflammatory processes tend to cause sudden visual loss.
- Compressive lesions such as tumors tend to progress gradually.
- Features of papilledema include edema of the optic discs, dilated tortuous veins, splinter hemorrhages on the disc, exudates on the disc, obliteration of the disc cup, and absent venous pulsations.

- Venous pulsations disappear when the cerebrospinal fluid (CSF) pressure is >210 mm of water. However, 20% of normal patients have no venous pulsations.
- Both papilledema and papillitis (inflammation of the optic disc or nerve) can cause visual loss, but this tends to occur earlier and be more severe in papillitis.

## Abnormal Eye Movements and Diplopia

Cranial nerves (CNs) III, IV, and VI control extraocular movements. One or more of these CNs can be affected and cause diplopia. Syndromes involving other cranial nerves are covered in Chapter 34.

- CN III palsy:
  - Patient notices diplopia (skew or vertical, sometimes horizontal) or ptosis.
  - Loss of CN III functions, including unilateral fixed and dilated pupil, extraocular movement abnormalities, and ptosis.
  - Differential diagnosis:
    Aneurysm (usually involves the posterior communicating artery).
    Uncal herniation syndrome.
    Midbrain lesion (ischemia, tumor, or stroke).
    Cavernous sinus lesions (also involves CN V-1 and V-2, IV and VI).
    Ischemia of CN III as in diabetes (usually is "pupil sparing").
    Leptomeningeal metastases.
- CN VI palsy:
  - Patient notices horizontal diplopia that is worse with distance vision and improves or corrects with near vision.
  - In unilateral lesions, the diplopia is worse when lateral gaze is attempted with the affected eye, improves at midposition, and resolves with gaze to the opposite side.
  - Differential diagnosis:
    Nonlocalizing (diplopia may be a nonlocalizing symptom).
    Increased intracranial pressure (ICP).
    Superior orbital fissure mass (also involves CNs III, IV, V-1).
    Cavernous sinus.
    Ischemia as in diabetes.
    Trauma.
    Pontine lesion.
    Leptomeningeal metastases.
- CN IV palsy:
  - Patient notices vertical diplopia.
  - Patient may have head tilt.

– Patient cannot move the affected eye down and in:

To diagnose CN IV palsy when in the presence of CN III palsy, ask the patient to look down and in. If CN IV is intact intorsion of that eye will occur.

– Differential diagnosis:

Trauma.

Pineal region mass.

Superior orbital fissure mass (also involves CNs III, $V_1$, VI).

Cavernous sinus.

- Nystagmus, named by the fast (corrective) component:
  - Downbeat nystagmus: lesions of the cervicomedullary junction.
  - Upbeat nystagmus: tumors of the cerebellum or medulla (e.g., medulloblastoma).
  - Lateral nystagmus: structural lesions or drugs.

## Abnormalities of the Pupil

- Horner's syndrome:
  - Unilateral small pupil, most noticeable in darkness (affected pupil fails to dilate normally in darkness).
  - Normal light and near reactions.
  - Ipsilateral ptosis.
  - Ipsilateral anhydrosis (loss of sweating).
  - Lesion of sympathetic innervation, usually apical lung mass or cervical paravertebral mass.
  - Pharmacologic testing can identify whether the Horner's syndrome is preganglionic or postganglionic.
- CN III palsy (unilateral fixed and dilated pupil, other features described previously).
- Tonic pupil (Adie's pupil: dilated pupil with minimal to no light reaction, but tonic constriction occurs with convergence):
  - Benign syndrome usually seen in young women, sometimes bilateral.
  - May be associated with depressed reflexes.

## Cortical Lesions

### Frontal Lobe Lesions

- The frontal lobe gaze center controls conjugate rapid voluntary eye movement (saccades) to the contralateral side.
- Destructive lesion: contralateral saccades impaired and eyes deviate toward the frontal lesion.
- Irritative lesion (i.e., seizures): eyes look away from lesion.

## Occipital Lesions

- The occipital gaze center controls voluntary tracking (pursuit) movements toward the ipsilateral side.
- Destructive lesions: pursuit movements toward the side of the lesion are jerky, usually associated with hemianopsia contralateral to the lesion.

## Pontine Lesions

- The pontine lateral gaze center controls ipsilateral horizontal gaze in response to vestibular and proprioceptive input.
- Destructive lesion: eyes look away from side of lesion.

# VII

## Pain and Terminal Care

# 53

# Palliative and Terminal Care

*Participation in this process challenges the clinician's emotional resources and medical skills. There is, however, the potential for professional satisfaction in helping to orchestrate a "good death," because the relief of suffering is at the very heart of medicine.*

—Kathleen Foley, 1997

## Overview and Philosophy

Despite significant advances in the diagnosis and treatment of primary and metastatic brain tumors and neurologic complications of cancer, most patients ultimately die of their tumors. The medical, social, and spiritual needs of dying neuro-oncology patients are similar to those of other cancer patients. However, due to the nature of their disease, they may be especially concerned about loss of cognitive functions and control of final care decisions. The terminal phase presents a significant challenge for patients and their caregivers. Physicians play a critical role in coordinating care for the dying patient and can foster a cohesive multidisciplinary approach that meets the individual needs of each patient and their loved ones.

Health care providers involved in the care of dying cancer patients must be prepared to guide the patient and family through the entire dying process. They must manage the anticipated physical and emotional symptoms that occur during the dying process. Furthermore, to provide effective care for the patient, they must cope appropriately with their own emotional, ethical, and spiritual issues about dying. Information about planning end-of-life care and appropriate references are provided here. Chapter 54 specifically covers pain management.

## Palliative Care

*Palliative care* is defined by the World Health Organization as "the active *total* care of patients whose disease is not responsive to curative treatment. Control of pain, of other symptoms, and of psychological, social, and spiritual problems is paramount. The goal of palliative care is achievement of the best quality of life for patients and their families."

The term *palliative care* generally is used to refer to patient care after tumor-specific therapy is stopped and the primary goal of treatment is to provide relief of symptoms and maintain function. Patients with incurable malignancies but who are not imminently dying can derive great benefit from high-quality palliative care.

## Terminal Care

The term *terminal care* generally refers to the care of patients who are expected to die within a short time, although there is no uniformly accepted definition of the specific time frame. Recent evidence suggests that physician's predictions of life expectancy often are incorrect, with a significant proportion of patients dying sooner or later than predicted. In the terminal phase, the primary goals of care are maintaining patient comfort and preparing the patient and loved ones for the patient's death. During this phase, the underlying disease as well as the side effects of medications used to alleviate symptoms often compromise the patient's ability to function.

## Avoiding Professional and Family Caregiver Burnout

Despite increasing recognition that providing competent care for the dying is a valuable and legitimate endeavor, the risk of caregiver burnout is high. For family caregivers, the physical, psychological, and emotional toll of caring for a dying loved one is more than most people can tolerate. An extensive support system and the opportunity to take respites are essential. Strategies for avoiding caregiver burnout are provided here, and the sources in the Suggested Reading section provide further information. Caregivers should be

- Familiar with ethical and medical guidelines regarding the care of dying patients.
- Prepared with strategies to address common symptoms with support by appropriate individuals and services for situations that they cannot readily manage.
- Engaged in regular activities to reduce stress: exercise, relaxation, spiritual, or religious practice.

- Able to foster a support system among caring professionals as well as an "external" support system from family and friends.

## Guidelines

The following guidelines are provided regarding the rights of physicians and patients during the dying process.

### Patient Rights

Every patient has the right to a dignified and appropriate death, including

- Medical care that is reliable, consistent with their wishes, and non-invasive, which involves adequate pain control and relief of distressing symptoms.
- Physical care that is timely, considerate, gentle, and reliable.
- Emotional care that is genuine and involved.
- Spiritual and religious care according to their desires.

Competent patients have the right to *self-determination* and therefore to refuse or terminate treatments. Patients do not have the right to request treatments that are illegal or medically unsound.

### Physician's Duties and Rights

- The physician has a duty to follow health care decisions competently made by his or her patients. Specifically, physicians have the duty to honor the competent patient's refusal of medical treatments.
- The physician has a duty to assist in decreasing suffering.
- The physician has a duty to transfer care to another physician if he or she is unable to comply with patient refusals or because of his or her own beliefs or knowledge base.
- The physician has a duty to actively solicit patient consent for treatments and interventions.
- The physician has a duty to educate the patient regarding treatment options and to solicit the patient's wishes while he or she still is competent.
- The physician has no obligation to promote death.
- The physician has no obligation to act against his or her own beliefs.
- The physician has no obligation to provide treatment that is medically unnecessary or unsound.
- The physician has no obligation to perform any act that is illegal.

## Planning End-of-Life Care

The following questions elicit decisions and plans that are important for planning end-of-life care for most patients. Some patients will have other needs and issues.

- Who will direct the patient's care?
- Where should terminal care occur: home, hospital, skilled nursing facility, inpatient hospice?
- Where does the patient wish to die? (This is not always the same as question 2.)
- Who does the patient want to be with? Who does the patient not want to be with?
- What does the patient want to do in the time remaining?
- Is there anywhere the patient wants to go before dying? Is this feasible?
- What financial concerns are there? Does the patient need assistance in settling affairs?
- What are the patient's religious and spiritual needs?
- What are the patient's advance directives?
- What are the symptoms that should be anticipated and prepared for?

When terminal care at home is chosen, the following specific issues need to be addressed:

- What hospice or home health services are available for the patient, and what can they provide? How often can someone come? Is someone available at all times?
- Who will be the primary caregiver? Who will provide assistance? Who will monitor and purchase medications?
- Who will be responsible for communicating with professional caregivers?
- Who will be the spokesperson to communicate with other loved ones?
- What is the contingency plan if the home situation becomes unsatisfactory? For example, if symptoms are uncontrollable or if the caregivers become weary, unreliable, or need to be away for a period of time?
- What should the caregivers do at the time of death? Who should they call (not 911), what funeral home will be used? A letter given to the family in advance for the police describing the patient's illness and that death is expected and due to natural causes can facilitate this step.

Issues regarding inpatient terminal care include:

- Can the facility provide adequate care, manage symptoms, and obtain medications?
- Does the facility have adequate physician and nursing support?

- How does the facility document, monitor, and follow the patient's advance directives?
- Is the facility close, so that family and friends can visit?
- Can the facility provide privacy for the patient?
- Who should the facility call when death is near?
- What funeral home should be used?

## Physician-Assisted Suicide and Euthanasia

Active public and medical debate continue regarding the ethics, morality, and medical issues surrounding physician-assisted suicide and euthanasia. Definitions for these terms are provided here, as are references from recent publications. No recommendations regarding the ethics or logistics of these measures are made. Rather, the focus of this chapter (and this book) has been toward providing competent, comprehensive, and compassionate care for the dying. Active, appropriate palliative care, which may inadvertently shorten life, does not constitute either euthanasia or physician-assisted suicide, rather it is good medical care.

*Physician-assisted suicide* occurs when the physician provides the necessary means for the patient to commit suicide, but death is not the direct result of the physician's action (physician assistance is not sufficient to accomplish suicide). For example, the physician prescribes a lethal dose of medication that the patient voluntarily ingests. This is illegal in all but one of the United States (Oregon).

*Voluntary active euthanasia* occurs when the physician accedes to the rational request of a competent patient and the physician directly causes the death of the patient. For example, the physician administers a known lethal dose of intravenous potassium chloride in response to a patient's request to end his or her life. This is considered an act of criminal homicide in the United States.

*Voluntary passive euthanasia* occurs when the physician abides by the rational refusal of treatment by a competent patient, knowing that the result will shorten the patient's life. For example, the physician terminates ventilatory support at the patient's request. This is accepted medical practice in the United States: physicians are morally and legally required to comply with a patient's request to refuse treatment.

## Suggested Reading

American Academy of Neurology Ethics and Humanities Subcommittee. Palliative care in neurology. *Neurology.* 1996;46(3):870–872.

Burt RA. The Supreme Court speaks. Not assisted suicide but a constitutional right to palliative care. *New Engl J Med.* 1997;337(17):1234–1236.

Cherny NI, Coyle N, Foley KM. Guidelines in the care of the dying cancer patient. *Hematol Oncol Clin North Am.* 1996;10(1):261–286.

Doyle D, Hanks GWC, MacDonald N (eds). *Oxford Textbook of Palliative Medicine.* New York: Oxford University Press, 1993.

Foley KM. Competent care for the dying instead of physician-assisted suicide. *N Engl J Med.* 1997;336(1);54–58.

Kashiwagi T. Psychosocial and spiritual issues in terminal care. *Psychiatry and Clin Neurosci.* 1995;49(suppl 1):S123–S127.

Mount BM. Volunteer support services, a key component of palliative care. *J Palliat Care.* 1992;8(1):59–64.

Voltz R, Borasio GD. Palliative therapy in the terminal stage of neurological disease. *J Neurol.* 1997;244(suppl 4):S2–S10.

Waller A, Caroline NL. *Handbook of Palliative Care* (2nd ed). Boston; Butterworth–Heinemann, 2000.

# 54

# Cancer Pain Management

## Overview and Significance

Significant pain occurs in at least one third of adults with cancer under active therapy and two thirds of patients with advanced cancer. For many patients, pain is the most frightening and disabling aspect of having cancer. Primary care physicians have an important role in cancer pain management because they often are the resource the patient relies on for pain management on an ongoing basis. A multidisciplinary team, led by a physician knowledgeable in pain management, is available at many of the larger cancer centers and serves as a valuable resource for patients and their physicians. Most patients derive great benefit from a comprehensive assessment by such a team. For example, a new lesion may be discovered that is amenable to specific treatment, specific causes of pain are defined, nonpharmacologic management options are explored, and psychosocial factors are identified including the diagnosis of major depression.

## Approach to the Patient

### Diagnosis

Effective pain management begins by delineating the type(s) of pain the patient is experiencing. Pain from more than one site or more than one etiology is common in cancer patients. A detailed history is critical and includes questions regarding the types and locations of pain, intensity of pain, how often pain is present, aggravating and alleviating factors, results of previous therapies, and ongoing chemotherapy or radiotherapy. Because pain occurs in the context of other distressing symptoms, such as anxiety, depression, insomnia, and nausea, these symptoms must be solicited by careful inquiry. Noncancer-related causes of pain that may have preceded the cancer diagnosis also are important to identify.

## Bone Pain

- Most common type of pain in cancer patients.
- Dull, aching, and well localized.
- May increase with movement but persists at rest.

## Visceral Pain

- Results from involvement of thoracic, abdominal, or pelvic visceral organs.
- Localization is vague.
- Certain movements may worsen the pain.
- Referral of pain to cutaneous sites may occur. Tenderness at the cutaneous sites may be found. For example, diaphragmatic pain refers to the shoulder and pelvic pain refers to the anterior or inner thighs.
- Type of pain is dull, squeezing, pressure sensation.
- Autonomic features are common when visceral pain is acute: diaphoresis, pallor, nausea, and vomiting.
- A general sense of distress or anxiety is common with visceral pain and may be the initial manifestation, particularly in patients already on analgesic agents.

## Neuropathic Pain

- Mild to severe.
- Character often is described as burning, dysesthetic, vise-like, shooting, "hot-poker," electric-shock sensations.
- Associated sensory loss may be present.
- Touching the affected areas may trigger pain but movement per se does not significantly worsen the pain. Patients may seek relief by changing positions, pacing, or rubbing unaffected body parts.
- Response to opiates is incomplete ("takes the edge off") and adjuvant treatment is critical.
- Dexamethasone may provide acute relief and should be used intravenously when severe pain is present (although less effective in postherpetic neuralgia).

## Pain Unrelated to Cancer

Common causes of such pain include peripheral neuropathy, osteoporosis, osteoarthritis, and lumbar disc disease. Migraine and other benign headache syndromes should be considered as contributing causes of headaches, particularly in younger patients.

## Comprehensive Management

Pain management should begin during the diagnostic process, and in some cases, diagnostic tests need to be deferred pending adequate pain control. Diagnostic testing should be performed as indicated to determine the exact nature of pain or to diagnose metastatic lesions or other pathology. Specific diagnosis may lead to primary treatment that may be more effective than analgesics in controlling pain. The most common example is the use of focal radiotherapy for bone pain. A comprehensive approach to cancer pain management includes

- Primary treatment with radiotherapy or chemotherapy when appropriate.
- Opiate and nonopiate analgesics.
- Management of associated symptoms, such as depression.
- Management of side effects, such as sedation and constipation.
- Nonpharmacologic management, including physical therapy, or relaxation training.
- Specialized anesthesia techniques, such as nerve blocks.
- Specialized neurosurgical interventions.

## Pharmacologic Approach

The World Health Organization Cancer Pain Relief Program has popularized the use of an "analgesic ladder" approach:

- Mild to moderate pain: nonopioid analgesic agents, such as acetaminophen and ibuprofen. If pain is uncontrolled, opioid analgesics are instituted (Table 54-1).
- Mild to moderate pain not responding to nonopioids: propoxyphene, oxycodone, and codeine in combination with nonopioid analgesics (Table 54-2).
- Moderate to severe pain: oxycodone at higher doses, morphine, hydromorphone, levorphanol, and oxymorphone.
  - Morphine and oxycodone are considered the opiate of choice for chronic oral use and are available in a wide variety of preparations including long-acting forms (see Table 54-1).
  - Meperidine is avoided because the accumulation of toxic metabolites can cause central nervous system (CNS) irritability, including seizures.
  - Narcotic partial agonists and mixed agonist-antagonists have no role in cancer pain management.

There is strong evidence for the effectiveness and dosing strategies associated with opiate analgesic use; however, use of some of the "adjunctive" (nonopiate) medications is empiric and dosing is based on use in other disease states.

**Table 54-1**   Selected Opioid Analgesics and Dosing

| Agent | Route | Starting Dose (opiate naïve patient) | Dose Range | Indications and Comments |
|---|---|---|---|---|
| **Weak opiates** | | | | |
| Propoxyphene | PO | Standardized pill sizes | | Increases carbamazepine levels |
| Codeine | PO | 10–30 mg q 4–6 hr | 30–60 mg q 4–6 h | Avoid doses >60 mg; move to strong opiate if ineffective |
| | PO | Acetaminophen/codeine tablet #3 = 500/30 | 1–2 tablets q 4–6 h | Avoid doses >60 mg; move to strong opiate if ineffective |
| **Strong opiates** | | | | |
| Morphine | PO | 5–10 mg q 2–3 h | Increase by 5 mg increments; available in liquid and tablets | Concentrated liquid formulation absorbed in oral mucosa; useful if swallowing is poor |
| | IM | 10 mg q 2–3 h | Increase by 2–4 mg per dose | Prefer subcutaneous route for comfort |
| | SC | 15 mg q 2-3 h | Increase by 5 mg increments | |
| | IV | 2–5 mg q 1–2 h | Increase by 2–4 mg per dose; consider continuous IV infusion; consider patient-controlled analgesia | Most effective route for acute pain management and rapid dose titration |

| Drug | Route | Dose | Titration | Comments |
|---|---|---|---|---|
| Controlled release morphine | PO | 10–20 mg q 8–12 h | Increase by 10 mg/dose increments every 3 days | Not effective for acute pain relief |
| Oxycodone | PO | 5–10 mg q 4–6 h | Increase by 5–10 mg increments | Available in combination with or without acetaminophen |
| Controlled release oxycodone | PO | 10 mg bid | Increase by 10–20 mg increments every 2–3 d | Not effective for acute pain relief |
| Hydromorphone | PO | 1–2 mg q 4–6 h | 2–4 mg q 4–6 h | Less pruritus than Morphine |
| | PR | 3 mg q 4–6 h | Increase by 3 mg increments | |
| Hydrocodone | PO | 30 mg q 4–6 h | 30–60 mg | Available combined with acetaminophen |
| Fentanyl transdermal system | Transdermal | Lowest patch: 25 µg/hr | Patches: 50 µg/hr, 75 µg/hr, 100 µg/hr Advance patch size q 3–6 days | Difficult to titrate, slow onset and action, slow decrease in dose after removing patch |
| Meperidine | IM | 50–75 mg q 4–6 h | 75–150 mg q 4 h | Not recommended; repeated administration can cause CNS toxicity including seizures |

PO, oral; IM, intramuscular; SC, subcutaneous; PR, rectal.

**Table 54-2** Selected Nonopioid Drugs for Management of Cancer Pain and Side Effects of Opiates

| Agent | Route | Starting Dose | Dose Range | Indications and Comments |
|---|---|---|---|---|
| **Analgesics** | | | | |
| Acetaminophen | PO | 650–1000 mg q 6h | Max: 4000 mg/d | Soft tissue and bone pain, potentiates affect of opiates, antipyretic |
| | PR | 1000 mg q 6 h | | |
| Aspirin | PO/PR | 650 mg q 4–6 h | Max: 4000 mg/d | Soft tissue and bone pain, antipyretic |
| **NSAIDs** | | | | |
| Ibuprofen | PO | 600–800 mg q 6h | Max: 2400 mg/d | Soft tissue and bone pain, headaches, better GI tolerance than aspirin |
| Naprosyn | PO | 250–500 mg q 12h | | As for Ibuprofen, longer acting |
| Ketorolac | PO | 10 mg q 6 h | | As for ibuprofen, parenteral use |
| | IM | 30–60 mg | Subsequent doses 15–30 mg q 6h or change to PO form | |
| **Steroids** | | | | |
| Dexamethasone | PO | 4–6 mg q 6 h | Total daily dose of 8–40 mg, may be divided bid to qid | Spinal cord compression, brain metastases, neuropathic pain, headaches, bone pain, anti-nausea effect, stimulates appetite |
| | IV | Same | Same as oral | Same as oral |
| Prednisone | PO | 10–40 mg q d | | Soft tissue and bone pain |
| **Anticonvulsants** | | | | |
| Carbamazepine | PO | 100–200 mg qd to bid, long acting formulation available | 400–2000, divided bid to tid, check serum levels at higher doses | Neuropathic pain, trigeminal neuralgia, paroxysmal nerve pain, start slowly for better GI tolerance |

| | | | |
|---|---|---|---|
| Gabapentin | PO | Increase by 100 mg increments every 3–4 days to reach 900–1800/d | Neuropathic pain, painful peripheral neuropathy |
| Phenytoin | PO/IV | 200–500/d, check serum levels | Neuropathic pain; limited effectiveness |
| Baclofen | PO | 5–10 mg bid to tid | Neuropathic pain, spasticity, hiccups, dose limited by sedation, start low dose and titrate slowly |
| Clonazepam | PO | 0.5–1.0 mg q 6–8 h | Most sedating anticonvulsant |
| **Antidepressants** | | | |
| Amitryptiline | PO | 10–25 mg qhs | Neuropathic pain, pain with anxiety/depressive component or insomnia, limited by cholinergic side effects |
| Nortriptiline | PO | 10–25 mg qhs | Similar to amitryptiline; less cholinergic side effects |
| **Stimulants** | | | |
| Methylphenidate | PO | 5 mg in A.M. | Helpful for opioid induced sedation, depression |
| Caffeine | PO | 40–80 mg q 6 h | Helpful for opioid induced sedation, rebound headache if stopped abruptly |
| **Antihistamines** | | | |
| Hydroxyzine | PO | 25 mg q 6h | Visceral pain, soft tissue pain, antiemetic, anti-anxiety |
| | IM | 25–100 mg | Same |

NSAIDs, nonsteroidal anti-inflammatory drugs; IV, intravenous; IM, intramuscular; PO, oral; PR, rectal; SC, subcutaneous; SL, sublingual; h, hour; mg, milligram; GI, gastrointestinal.

Most pain can be controlled acutely with opiates and anti-inflammatory agents. Patients with difficult pain syndromes require the empiric use of opiates and adjunctive medications in an organized sequence to identify medications and combinations that provide meaningful pain control with acceptable side effects.

## Opioids

The choice of agent is based on the severity of pain, desired route of treatment, and the patient's previous experience with opioid analgesics (see Table 49-1). The initial approach is to treat with a single agent and increase the dose until adequate analgesia is achieved or unmanageable side effects develop. Tolerance develops to some of the adverse side effects of opioids (e.g., respiratory sedation), whereas others are dose related (e.g., constipation). For most patients, sedation is the limiting side effect.

The following are some potential side effects of opiates and their management:

- Sedation and cognitive slowing:
  - Minimize by using long-acting compounds and discontinuing other medications with sedating effects.
  - Try adjunctive treatment with stimulant agents (methylphenidate).
- Constipation (see Chapter 33).
- Nausea and vomiting:
  - Add agents with antiemetic effect (see Chapter 46).
  - Change to a different opiate.
- Multifocal myoclonus occurs primarily with high doses of parenteral opiates. When this symptom is distressing to the patient or family, it can be attenuated with dose reduction (if tolerable) or by adding either benzodiazepines or barbiturates.
- Respiratory depression (see later).
- *Psychological dependence* ("addiction") refers to the use of opiates other than for pain control and is associated with craving and drug seeking behavior.
  - Addiction is rare in cancer patients. Unfortunately, the potential for addiction remains a common concern among cancer patients and some physicians.
  - Patients with a history of drug abuse should be carefully evaluated and medications monitored. The concern for readdiction should not interfere with the control of cancer pain.

Tolerance (physical dependence) develops in all patients taking chronic opiates. This makes the patient vulnerable to opiate withdrawal if the opiate is stopped abruptly, pharmacologically reversed with naloxone, or the dose is lowered significantly. Strategies to avoid the occurrence of withdrawal and its unpleasant symptoms include the following:

- If pain lessens due to treatment of underlying disease, taper off the opiate dose slowly.
- Patients on chronic oral opiates who become unable to take oral medications should be transferred to equivalent doses of parental opiates as quickly as possible.
- When patients are given intravenous opiates, the possibility of respiratory sedation including respiratory arrest should be discussed with the patient and caregivers in advance. Resuscitation with naloxone should be discussed and the patient's advance directives noted and adhered to. Mild respiratory depression often can be managed with continuous stimulation (to maintain the awake state) and lowering the dose of opiate. Diluted doses of naloxone (0.4 mg in 10 cc of NS) have been used successfully to reverse respiratory depression and avoid sudden withdrawal symptoms.

## *Nonopioids*

Selected nonopioid agents useful in cancer pain management are summarized in Table 54-2. Uses of adjunctive medications include

- Single-agent management of mild to moderate pain.
- Additive analgesia in combination with opioids.
- Attenuation of the side effects of opioids.
- Treatment of neuropathic pain.

## Suggested Reading

DeVita VT, Hellman S, Rosenberg SA. *Cancer: Principles and Practice of Oncology.* Philadelphia: J.B. Lippincott, 1993.

Foley KM. Advances in cancer pain. *Arch Neurol.* 1999;56(4):413–417.

MacFarlane BV, Wright A, O'Callaghan J, et al. Chronic neuropathic pain and its control by drugs. *Pharmacol Ther.* 1997;75(1):1–19.

Mount B. Morphine drips, terminal sedation, and slow euthanasia: Definitions and facts, not anecdotes. *J Palliat Care.* 1996;12(4):31–37.

Urba SG. Nonpharmacologic pain management in terminal care. *Clin Geriatr Med.* 1996;12(2):301–311.

World Health Organization. *Cancer Pain Relief.* Geneva: World Health Organization, 1986.

# APPENDIX I

# Resources for Patients and Physicians

These organizations provide a variety of information and services. Some are specifically directed toward brain tumor patients; others are more general in nature. These organizations also provide referrals to other groups that can assist with particular concerns.

## American Brain Tumor Association (ABTA)

2720 River Road, Des Plaines, IL 60018
Phone: 847-827-9910
Patient information: 1-800-886-2282
Fax: 847-827-9918
Website: www.abta.org
  – Summaries of treatment options, written in lay language.
  – No-cost basic information about brain tumors, as well as pamphlets about specific primary brain tumors and tumors that have metastasized to the brain.
  – Information about support groups, coping strategies, other psychosocial aspects of care, and fundraising efforts.
  – Names of physicians involved in clinical trials are available on request.
  – Newsletter, *Message Line*.

## American Cancer Society

National Office: 1599 Clifton Road Northeast, Atlanta, GA 30329-4251
Phone: 1-800-ACS-2345 (1-800-227-2345)
Website: www.cancer.org
  - Contact the national office to get information about local chapters.
  - Information provided in both English and Spanish.

## Angel Flight

3237 Donald Douglas Loop South, Santa Monica, CA 90405
Phone: 888-4-AN-ANGEL or 310-390-2958
24-hour emergency response phone: 310-456-2035
Fax: (310) 397-9636
Website: www.angelflight.org
  - Provides no-cost air transportation for treatment of medically stable patients via a network of private aircraft.
  - Serves the western United States.

## Association of Community Cancer Centers

11600 Nebel Street, Suite 201, Rockville, MD 20852
Phone: 301-984-9496
Fax: 301-770-1949
Website: www.accc-cancer.org
  - Geographic listing of community cancer centers.
  - Standards for cancer programs.
  - Updates on legislation and other political aspects of cancer.

## Brain Tumor Foundation of Canada

650 Waterloo Street, Suite 100, London, Ontario N6B 2R4
Phone: 1-800-265-5106 or 519-642-7755
Fax: 519-642-7192
Website: www.btfc.org
  - Guidebooks written for adults and parents of children with brain tumors.
  - Information about resources in Canada for brain tumor patients.
  - Information provided in both English and French.

## The Brain Tumor Society

124 Watertown Street, Suite 3H, Watertown, MA 02472
Phone: 800-770-TBTS (8287)
Fax: 617-924-9998
Website: www.tbts.org
 – Emphasis on quality of life, education, psychosocial support.
 – Supports scientific research projects and clinical care, primarily in the northeastern United States.

## Cancer Care

275 Seventh Avenue, New York, NY 10001
Phone: 1-800-813-HOPE (4673) or 212-302-2400
Fax: 212-719-0263
Website: www.cancercare.org
 – Social service organization aimed at implementing their philosophy that "life does not end when cancer begins."
 – The toll free number connects the user to help with a wide variety of practical and psychosocial problems.
 – The website includes information, including nationwide resources, when the need is less urgent.
 – An on-line "library" of cancer-related materials and media reports. Cancer Care also conducts "teleconferences," which are educational programs conducted via conference call, including several focused on brain tumors.
 – All services are free.

## Centerwatch

22 Thomson Place, 36T1, Boston, MA 02210-1212
Phone: 617-856-5900
Fax: 617-856-5901
Website: www.centerwatch.com
 – Listings of active clinical trials state-by-state and worldwide.
 – Profiles of centers that have chosen to list their studies on this web site.
 – Current listings for brain tumors including academic medical centers, industry-sponsored trials, and private clinical research organizations.
 – Patients may sign up for a notification service that provides ongoing information about newly activated clinical trials.

## Children's Brain Tumor Foundation

274 Madison Avenue, Suite 1301, New York, NY 10016
Phone: 212-448-9494
Fax: 212-448-1022
Website: www.cbtf.org
  - Advocacy, education, and psychosocial support on behalf of children diagnosed with a brain tumor.
  - Family Outreach Project and Parent-to-Parent Network provide a range of services for families and brain tumor survivors.

## Choice in Dying

475 Riverside Drive, Room 1852, New York, NY 10115
Phone: 1-800-989-WILL (9455) or 212-870-2003
Fax: 212-870-2040
Website: www.choices.org
  - Focus on end-of-life issues: medical, legal psychosocial. Offers guidebooks, counseling line.

## Clinical Trials and Noteworthy Treatments for Brain Tumors

1100 Peninsula Blvd., Hewlett, NY 11557
Phone: 516-295-4740
Fax: 516-295-2870
Website: www.virtualtrials.com
  - Listing of active brain tumor clinical trials throughout the world.
  - The Musella Foundation for Brain Tumor Research and Information maintains this website. The foundation also coordinates the Brain Tumor Virtual Study, a database of information provided by any brain tumor patient who signs informed consent and submits his or her medical records.

## Corporate Angel Network

Westchester County Airport, 1 Loop Road, White Plains, NY 10604
Phone: 914-328-1313
Website: www.corpangelnetwork.org
  - Organization that makes it possible for medically stable patients to obtain free flights on corporate aircraft to travel to treatment centers.

## International Cancer Alliance

4853 Cordell Avenue, Suite 206, Bethesda, MD 20814
Phone: 1-800-ICARE-61 or 301-654-7933
Fax: 301-654-8684
Website: www.icare.org
  – Provides a Cancer Therapy Review via e-mail, fax, or mail with information about diagnosis, treatment, and clinical trials for brain tumors (free of charge, although donations are requested to cover costs).
  – Electronic bulletin board on which notices of events, availability of publications, and requests for information can be "posted."

## National Brain Tumor Foundation (NBTF)

414 13th Street, Suite 700, Oakland, CA 94612
Phone: 510-839-9777
Patient Information: 1-800-934-CURE (2873)
Fax: 510-839-9779
Website: http://www.braintumor.org
  – Answers to general questions about diagnosis and treatment of brain tumors, written in lay language.
  – Information guides about brain tumors, support groups, and resources (including resources for and the NBTF newsletter, *Search*) can be requested.
  – Extensive links to other websites and general cancer-related information.

## National Cancer Institute (NCI)

National Institutes of Health, Bethesda, MD 20892
  – Cancer Information Service (the NCI telephone information service): Phone: 1-800-4-CANCER (1-800-422-6237)
  – Cancernet (the NCI cancer information website): Website: http://cancernet.nci.nih.gov
  – Cancermail (the NCI's information electronic mail address, include the word *help* in the body of the message): Website: cancermail@cips.nci.nih.gov
  – Cancerfax (the NCI fax information line): Phone: 1-800-624-2511 or 301-402-5874
  – All these resources provide access to clinical trial listings, genetics, and screening information, supportive care information.
  – Information provided in both English and Spanish.

## National Coalition for Cancer Survivorship

1010 Wayne Avenue, Suite 770, Silver Spring, MD 20910
Phone: 877-NCCS-YES (622-7937) or 301-650-9127
Fax: 301-565-9670
Website: www.cansearch.org
- Emphasis on practical and psychosocial cancer survivorship issues, including discrimination and legal problems.
- Information provided in both English and Spanish.

## National Hospice and Palliative Care Organization

1700 Diagonal Road, Suite 300, Alexandria, VA 22314
Phone: 703-837-1500
Fax: 703-525-5762
Website: www.nhpco.org
- Provides information about alternatives for end-of-life care and caregiving.

## National Society of Genetic Counselors

233 Canterbury Drive, Wallingford, PA 19086
Phone: 610-872-7608
Website: www.nsgc.org
- The professional organization of genetic counselors.
- This site may be of particular interest to those with more than one family member with a brain tumor.

## Oncolink

Website: http://cancer.med.upenn.edu
- A website with a focus on education and information dissemination.
- Citations, abstracts of articles in a wide variety of medical journals; selected cancer-related articles in newspapers and popular magazines; links to other cancer-related websites.
- Information about financial and psychosocial issues.
- Information about clinical trials, including those at the University of Pennsylvania, which maintains this site.

## Oncology Nursing Society

501 Holiday Drive, Pittsburgh, PA 15220
Phone: 412-921-7373
Fax: 412-921-6565
Website: www.ons.org
- The professional organization of nurses who specialize in oncology.
- Information about treatment options, symptom management, survivorship, and palliative care.
- Focus on cancer-related fatigue, with special website on this topic: www.cancerfatigue.org.

# APPENDIX II

# Karnofsky Performance Status

| KPS % | Karnofsky Score |
|-------|-----------------|
| 100 | Normal; no complaints; no evidence of disease |
| 90 | Able to carry out normal activity; minor signs or symptoms of disease |
| 80 | Normal activity with effort; some signs or symptoms of disease |
| 70 | Cares for self; unable to carry on normal activity or do active work |
| 60 | Requires occasional assistance but is able to care for most needs |
| 50 | Requires considerable assistance and frequent medical care |
| 40 | Disabled; requires special care and assistance |
| 30 | Severely disabled; hospitalization indicated, but death not imminent |
| 20 | Very sick; hospitalization necessary; active support treatment necessary |
| 10 | Moribund; fatal processes progressing rapidly |
| 0 | Dead |

# Index